Lessons Learned

Stroke Recovery
From a Caregiver's Perspective

D0873614

Berenice E. Kleiman

Cleveland Clinic Press

Cleveland, Ohio

Lessons Learned
Stroke Recovery From a Caregiver's Perspective

Cleveland Clinic Press

Contact:
Cleveland Clinic Press
9500 Euclid Avenue NA32 • Cleveland, Ohio 44195 • 216-445-5547
delongk@ccf.org • www.clevelandclinicpress.org

This book is not intended to replace personal medical care and supervision; there is no substitute for the information and experience that your doctor can provide. Rather, it is our hope that this book will provide additional information to help people understand the nature of stroke and stroke recovery.

Proper medical care should always be tailored to the individual patient. If you read something in this book that seems to conflict with your doctor's instructions, contact your doctor to discuss your questions. Because each individual case differs, there may be good reasons for an individual's treatment to differ from the information presented in this book. If you have any questions about any treatment mentioned in this book, consult your doctor.

Kleiman, Berenice, 1937-
Lessons Learned: Stroke Recovery From a Caregiver's Perspective
Berenice E. Kleiman.
p. cm.
Sequel to: *One Stroke, Two Survivors.* 2006.
Includes bibliographical references and index.
ISBN 978-1-59624-007-0 (alk. paper)
1. Kleiman, Herb. 2. Kleiman, Berenice, 1937-
3. Cerebrovascular disease–Popular works.
4. Cerebrovascular disease–Patients–Rehabilitation–Popular works.
5. Cerebrovascular disease–Patients–Family relationships–Popular works.
I. Kleiman, Berenice, 1937- *One Stroke, Two Survivors.* II. Title.
RC388.5.K5745 2007
616.8'103–dc22   2007006721

Book design by Kathy Dunasky

To Herb,

My husband and hero!

Contact Berenice Kleiman at:

www.onestroketwosurvivors.com

berenice@onestroketwosurvivors.com

herb@onestroketwosurvivors.com

Contents

Preface

Stroke strikes without warning. It can hit the most unsuspecting with strange, awful randomness. Delay in recognizing the signs and seeking emergency medical treatment worsens the outcome and often leads to life-changing consequences. Although most families in the U.S. will eventually deal with stroke, misinformation is widespread.

Ask three out of four nonmedical people to name even one sign of stroke and they will respond with a blank stare or simply shake their heads. Unlike heart disease and cancer, the other leading causes of death, stroke lurks in the shadows. People justify their avoidance on a series of miscalculations that stroke won't happen to them. Or, if it does, it will kill them immediately, so why worry?

Ten Deadly Myths about Stroke

Myth 1. Stroke happens to other people.
Don't fool yourself. Stroke is widespread and ranks just behind heart disease and cancer as the third leading cause of death in the U.S. Stroke is also the leading cause of serious, long-term disability in the United States.

Myth 2. Stroke is a Medicare malady, so if I'm not "of age," why should I worry?
Do be concerned for yourself as well as your parents and grandparents: 28 percent of people who suffer a stroke in a given year are under age 65.

Myth 3. With no previous family history of stroke, my spouse and I are safe.

Stroke doesn't necessarily follow genetic lines. People with arteriosclerosis and diabetes carry greater risk. But any condition, known or silent, that creates either clotting or massive bleeding potentially can affect the brain. Each year, about 700,000 people suffer a stroke. About 500,000 of these are first attacks, and 200,000 are recurrent attacks.

Myth 4. You'll know immediately when you or a loved one has a stroke.

Fewer than 20 percent of stroke sufferers and their spouses recognize the early signs of stroke. Too many mistakenly believe that a sudden severe headache, numbness or paralysis, dizziness, or a balance problem will become self-correcting after a nap or a good night's sleep.

Myth 5. You have a three- or four-hour window to get to an emergency room.

Stroke is a medical emergency and requires prompt action to arrest brain damage. Valuable hours can be lost in an emergency room waiting for treatment. Act quickly and responsibly to seek help.

Myth 6. EMS teams and hospitals are knowledgeable and will act quickly.

It is your responsibility to recognize the signs of stroke and flag these as soon as you call EMS or choose a hospital. Local rules often require paramedics to rush a patient to the nearest hospital, without regard to expertise. Not all EMS teams or hospitals are trained to recognize stroke and provide emergency treatment for patients. Not all hospitals offer the wide range of technical expertise to break up clots or provide immediate surgery to remove clotted blood in the brain following a cerebral hemorrhage. Much time can be lost.

Myth 7. Once you've had a stroke, your life is over.

Levels of mortality are decreasing as medical science develops improved means to open blocked arteries more promptly. About 4.7 million stroke survivors (2.3 million men, 2.4 million women) who benefit from these advanced technologies are alive today. Some strokes are minimal and leave few outward signs. Those with more massive deterioration require physical, occupational, and speech therapies to reestablish movement and communication. A rehab psychologist can also be a valuable member of your team.

Myth 8. The health of only the stroke victim is affected.

Not so. Almost one-half of stroke survivors rely on family caregivers to assist them with the physical, cognitive, behavioral, and emotional changes commonly associated with stroke. In excess of 50 million people provide care for a chronically ill, disabled, or aged family member or friend during any given year. Family caregivers who provide care for 36 or more hours weekly are more likely than noncaregivers to experience symptoms of depression or anxiety. For spousal caregivers, the rate is six times higher.

Myth 9. The best solution for the stroke survivor is a permanent nursing home.

No two strokes are alike. This decision depends upon the severity of the stroke, condition of the spouse or other family caregiver (physical as well as financial), and availability of therapies and rehab support. With persistent hard work, commitment, and determination, survivors of massive strokes that affect movement and communication are capable of improvement.

Myth 10. The patient and his/her family should accept, not question, medical care.

Most patients, particularly those with complications that often follow stroke and other forms of chronic illness, benefit from a second opinion and another perspective, preferably from a board-certified specialist in a different medical system. The Internet offers a vast array of medical information and allows you to research your medical malady, e.g., stroke and facial pain. While you will not qualify as a medical specialist, you can familiarize yourself with current and possibly promising new studies.

My husband Herb is the survivor of a massive stroke. Herb was unable to differentiate his minor symptoms from other ongoing medical problems. He went to sleep that eventful first night without sharing his concerns with me, basically hoping he'd feel better in the morning. By the time I heard his slurred words and sought help many hours later, clots were already in motion, blocking vital arteries in his brain.

Herb often tells others that "we were zero prepared" for stroke. Actually his timing was in our favor. At 66, he was under Medicare's protective umbrella. His excellent insurance supplement is the most inclusive available in our state. Had we been truly unprepared, medical and rehabilitation costs alone would have wiped out our savings.

On the other hand, Herb's long-term disability has taken a profound emotional toll on both of us. Following his stabilization and lengthy rehab program, Herb and I willed ourselves to push his limiting boundaries and improve his quality of life. Our efforts are continuing but not always successful because of numerous secondary complications, depression, and diminished energy on both our parts. Herb sometimes slips backward.

But in aggregate, and through great effort by those on our team and us, my husband is making amazing progress. He has regained recognizable speech and sharpens his damaged conceptual reasoning with crossword puzzles, outside cultural programs, and articles and e-mails that he writes on a word processor. Paralyzed on his right side, Herb walks with a pyramid walker that he grips in his left hand. I hold his gait belt and supervise. Setbacks when we least expect them are part of this post-stroke life to which we must both adjust.

For me, the caregiver's learning curve was exceptionally difficult. Even after six years, I still run into emotional buzz saws. Strokes can repeat. In order for Herb to maintain good cardiovascular conditioning, he must actively exercise at home and at a fitness center. Sometimes we get tired of the grind and the constant exercise regimen. Playing hooky once in a while helps us to feel that we are not programmed robots. But we return to the regimen because stroke and other long-term disabilities tolerate no passive positions. To stop means to slide backward.

It's hard to view the effects of stroke and feel grateful. We miss our former lives, our careers, and our independence. Yet we've demonstrated the fallacy of an early medical assertion that my husband would probably wind up in a nursing home with a feeding tube. Both of us recognize that we have come very far, although on a relative scale it is certainly not as far as we'd prefer.

Shortly after finishing our book, *One Stroke, Two Survivors*, I received a call from a woman who asked for my advice. Her husband had suffered a massive stroke several months earlier. Among the 20 percent of stroke victims under 50, he suffers from both paralysis and aphasia. His health insurance had reached its maximum and the inpatient rehabilitation facility chose to discharge him immediately.

The caller was caught in a terrible dilemma, forced to decide whether to place her husband in a nursing home permanently or care for him at home. She was unable to provide around-the-clock nursing care by herself because their young children needed the income and security provided by her full-time position. Adding to the pressure of this decision-making process was her feeling that she was totally unprepared to be a caregiver.

Advice on whether to become a caregiver is not something that one person, particularly a stranger, can offer another. It is altogether too personal and the implications it imposes run too deep. I could only listen with quiet empathy and suggest various community resources that might professionally help her to evaluate her options.

The caregiver choice is incredibly difficult. Spousal and family members who become caregivers must put their own lives and needs on hold as they tackle responsibilities for which they have little or no training. Making a decision for home over custodial care involves many factors. Key among these are the relationship of the patient to the caregiver, the health of each, economic realities, and whether they share a profound commitment to work together toward improvement. The success factor diminishes when one or more of these factors is missing on the part of either.

Myopic medical advice too often discourages potential caregivers. Specialists who deal with the early stages of stroke are unaware of the progress that some survivors make further down the road. Advice they repeatedly give to family members, stating that stroke survivors have a window of only three to six months to improve, is blatantly wrong, ratchets up unnecessary pressure, and can contribute to a poor outcome.

Six years ago, in the face of negative professional advice, I chose to bring my husband home and care for him myself. For us it was the right decision. Because there was available so little practical information about home care for a stroke survivor with his many needs, the process was very difficult. Through my own hardheadedness, helpful advice from others, and simple luck, I muddled through a range of complicated problems.

Although my husband's recovery is an ongoing process, we continue to make progress. It required challenging the medical system to become more responsive to my husband's needs and searching for specialists and therapists willing to support our efforts. I discarded the others. There is simply no room for negative or indifferent professionals.

Lessons Learned shares simple, everyday solutions to chronic and long-term disability problems that work for us. It also looks at these demands through the eyes and needs of a caregiver. I encourage you to adapt what you need to meet your own special needs.

The biggest message my husband and I can share with you is one of hope. With persistent hard work and determination, all things are possible!

Berenice E. Kleiman
April, 2007

Chapter 1
The Beginning
Strokes Happen

Hindsight is always 20/20, and many of us later reflect on clues we probably missed: wispy handwriting, a strange headache, perhaps a stumble the day before. Stroke is often camouflaged in the guise of many lesser maladies. Some victims experience severe headaches or paralysis, but these unmistakable occurrences are less frequent. More often, clots that block major arteries in the neck and brain emerge only with a slight headache, slurring of words, sudden dizziness, numbness of a limb, or loss of balance.

Because of these subtle early stages, most people completely miss the two- to three-hour window to gain a clot-breaking injection that can restore critical blood flow. Instead, until it is stabilized, the stroke glides across major sections of the brain and blocks the flow of oxygen. Brain tissue that controls voluntary and involuntary functions is destroyed.

The high cost of medical care and inflexible health-care insurance policies discourage many of us from running to an emergency room with "minor" symptoms or false alarms. We're legitimately afraid to incur a huge bill, a long wait, and probably a casual dismissal. Even in the emergency room, we sit patiently for hours waiting our turn. Once stroke settles in, the effects are unmistakable…and irreversible. But you can fight back!

Lessons Learned

Learn about stroke, preferably in advance.

There are two types of strokes. The first occurs when the blood supply to part of the brain is suddenly interrupted by a blood clot. The second, when a blood vessel in the brain bursts, pouring blood into the spaces surrounding brain cells. Symptoms are similar and appear suddenly. Often more than one symptom can be present at the same time.

The most important risk factors for stroke are hypertension, heart disease, diabetes, and smoking. Statistically, men have a higher risk for stroke than women, and men have strokes earlier in life.

Recognize the first signs of stroke.

- Numbness or paralysis in the face, arm, or leg, commonly on one side of the body
- Loss of vision
- Loss or slurring of speech
- Sudden severe headache
- Balance or coordination problem
- Dizziness
- Loss of consciousness

Seek medical help immediately.

It is imperative if you experience red-flag symptoms that you call 911 immediately. Use of tPA, the injection that breaks up blood clots, can

...nimize the risk of subsequent stroke-related paralysis or death if it used within the first three hours. Beyond that limited window, the medication can have a harmful effect and precipitate massive bleeding in the brain.

Fewer than 15 percent of stroke victims recognize initial signs of their stroke and seek treatment within three hours. Fewer still, not even 7 percent of stroke patients admitted to the hospital, receive clot-busting drugs. Most people in circumstances similar to my husband's go to bed hoping that sleep alone will improve their situation. Even if you are confused or unsure about the gravity of the symptoms, you must get to a hospital while these drugs can be effective. Stroke is a medical emergency!

State your suspicion of stroke up front.

Not all EMS squads or hospitals are trained to deal with stroke. When you dial 911, you must state your suspicion of stroke up front. Request an emergency crew and a hospital trained to handle tPA. Some communities have rules requiring EMS to take the victim to the nearest hospital regardless of its qualifications. You must be assertive. The faster you reach proper emergency support, the less brain destruction will result. Scout in advance and become familiar with the tertiary care stroke centers in your area.

Don't count on a three- to four-hour margin for action.

Don't believe, as I did, that you have a protective window of three to four hours to seek help. Medical authorities have recently revised this directive downward to two to three hours. Also, you must allow for precious time that can often be lost in the emergency room while you register and wait for help. If you believe your loved one is showing signs of stroke and the time is within the crucial window, state this up front and insist upon immediate care.

Carry a cell phone and prepaid telephone card.

Be sure you add vital medical and family phone numbers to the speed dial, keep your cell phone well charged, and carry it at all times. We wasted unnecessary time stopping at home to call our physician because I had neither his phone number nor a phone readily available. A prepaid telephone card comes in handy in health-care institutions where you must turn off the cell phone. It is also a good gift to ask others to bring when you are already in the hospital.

Alert family members and/or friends as soon as possible.

It is devastating to be alone during times of crisis. The support of family and friends can be comforting during long periods as you await results from medical and surgical procedures. Pragmatically, you may also need to call upon the medical expertise or advocacy of someone close to you who can translate medical terms and advise about the risks of recommended procedures.

Invite collective prayer.

Collective prayer builds strength, creates great energy, and can move mountains. I have become a believer in its power. Urge family and friends to pray for you.

Remain as an advocate by the side of your loved one.

Emergency rooms and hospitals, whether large or small, are busy, impersonal, even frightening institutions. No one on staff has time to pay attention as closely as you can. Stay with your patient. Trust your instincts and spot problems early. Don't hesitate to call for help when necessary.

Keep a notebook.

Date and write down all medical explanations, instructions, observations, and areas of confusion or concern. Your notebook provides a well-organized tool for subsequent reference. If you or other family members monitor the patient in shifts, your notes will be available to the next shift and allow them to add their comments.

Chapter 2
Stabilizing
Nothing Is a Layup

A hospital is not a comforting environment. Hope and expectation are luxuries that the medical establishment can little afford. Often, perhaps because of our litigious environment, physicians and support staff are much too pressured to overpromise or discuss anything other than immediate patient care.

Much of what takes place either in the emergency room or on the floor is beyond the experience or understanding of family members. Medical lingo, often without translation, is difficult for lay people to understand, especially under life-or-death pressure. Although staff social workers and members of the clergy are usually available, family members must formally request their support.

Once the patient is stabilized, next steps may include transfer to either a long-term nursing home or a rehabilitation facility. The choice between custodial care and sustained rehabilitation leads in distinctly different directions. Family members may find the advice of staff members (nurses as well as physicians) helpful in choosing a transfer facility. Since specialists see only one part of the recovery spectrum, the caregiver's decision may run counter to prevailing medical advice.

In our case, we ignored the dire prediction that my husband would probably wind up in a nursing home with a feeding tube. "Hell, no!" was my response. Although Herb had right-side paralysis (hemiplegia) and could barely hold up his head, walk, talk, or swallow, I had little doubt that he would improve. He simply had to. Our son and I vowed that we would do everything in our power to make sure that he did. We did, he did, and that made all the difference!

Lessons Learned

Check for a facility that can accommodate family members who want to stay overnight.

Hospitals often have small lounges tucked away for family members of patients in intensive and critical care. The nurse's station may also issue hospital blankets upon request should you plan to remain overnight.

Remember that encouragement can be found everywhere.

Physicians and nurses are trained to provide basic facts and little else. Sometimes hope can appear in the form of a smile, an act of kindness, or even a thoughtful word from a stranger.

Research your next steps.

After a patient is stabilized, there is usually rehab. Keep the process moving. In a metropolitan area you may have choices. Consider your options: whether you prefer an aggressive program or one geared more toward maintenance. The hospital social worker should have information to assist in your decision but, if possible, also ask the medical staff and friends for their recommendations. Accessibility is also a significant factor, should you plan to make daily visits. And, of course, cost is critical and may or may not be covered by your health-care insurance.

Be sure the ambulance driver knows the way.

Assume nothing. In case your ambulance driver gets lost on the way to the rehab facility, be sure you have your own directions in hand.

Chapter 3
The Rehab Hospital
Getting Down to Work

Rehab hospitals offer two basic components: nursing care and rehab therapies. Much like the training routines at boot camp, a continuing series of therapies fills most of the daily program. Physical therapists (PT) initiate a series of demanding exercises to help patients restore functional mobility. Occupational therapists focus on basic motor functioning (primarily involving the upper torso) and basic tasks to ease the patient back into the everyday home environment. Speech therapists help to shape thoughts, transform ideas into words, and strengthen the face and neck muscles that facilitate swallowing.

From the beginning, I requested that a rehab psychologist become part of our team. While other staff members would care for Herb's physical needs, the psychologist would help him adjust to his current and future post-stroke situation. We were fortunate to find an amazing professional, just right for my husband, who continues to work with both of us on new and recurring adjustment needs.

My biggest gripe concerned not the therapies but shortcomings in nursing care and caregiver training. Herb had use of only one side and needed a call button repositioned on his left. Food packets had to be opened for him, and he needed close surveillance on the toilet and in his wheelchair. An apparent lack of cooperation became a huge problem.

As a caregiver I needed training in tasks that I would have to do by myself later within the home environment. Although I requested help early in his program and defined my needs for instruction in toileting and learning how to bathe and dress Herb, move him from one seat to another, use his glucose monitor, and administer medications, much of the training came bunched together in the last week of rehab. There was too much for me to take in. I could have absorbed more had the training begun earlier and been divided into three or four sessions staggered through the entire rehab program. It would also have been helpful and practical to learn on equipment comparable to what I would later use at home. This is where hindsight can help others!

Lessons Learned

Check to see that the patient can readily reach emergency call buttons.

Make sure that both call button and telephone are positioned on your patient's usable side of the bed and readily accessible at all times.

Participate in therapies.

Participate in formal therapies both during sessions and in subsequent room exercises. Encouragement and practice are vital to your patient's rehab success. The program also readies the caregiver for independent home efforts that eventually follow.

Insist that the rehab hospital provide caregiver instruction.

When a disabled stroke victim returns home, family members are suddenly thrust, with little preparation, into new, highly stressful, and very dangerous roles as caregivers. Ask for a schedule for caregiver/home preparation. If they're not already planned, request at least four training sessions (forty-five-minute sessions are ideal) spread through the full course of the rehab program. Avoid bundling them into the final week. Also insist that your therapist team evaluate your home for wheelchair accessibility several weeks before discharge to allow you needed time to arrange adaptations.

Include a rehab psychologist as part of your recovery team.

Depression, a serious medical condition that affects thoughts and feelings, is often associated with abnormal functioning of the brain. Treatment for depression can shorten the rehabilitation process, lead to a more rapid recovery, and, in the long run, save health-care costs for both the patient and the insurance company. A rehab psychologist is trained to work with stroke patients and ease their functional adjustment both in rehab and back later into everyday life. Find one with whom both you and the stroke survivor are comfortable for the long term. The average duration of major depression in people who have suffered a stroke is just under a year.

Identify the hospital unit head or designated person in charge.

Request that the name and phone number of this unit head be positioned in a prominent location in your patient's room. Keep a dated record of derelictions in care and treatment. Report care that is negligent or below the standards of the Patient's Bill of Rights posted in your hospital room.

Propose a team progress meeting midway through the rehab program.

Ask to meet with the full medical team, including rehab specialist, psychologist, social worker, and therapists, to discuss the patient's progress and expectations. Do not allow the staff to delay this meeting until immediately before discharge. Think through and prepare a detailed list of your questions.

Chapter 4

The 24-Hour Furlough

When You Think You've Reached the Lowest Level of Hell, Watch Out for the Next Descent

Our rehab hospital uses a twenty-four-hour "trial" to measure whether families feel competent to assume the full responsibility for their incapacitated patient. Herb's leave came only four days before final discharge and less than one week after his therapists had made a home visit and declared our home thoroughly inaccessible. The nurses decreed in that last week that it was finally time to teach me how to care for my husband's many complex medical needs.

Unfortunately, everything hit the fan at one time. I had to order and oversee installation of miscellaneous home medical equipment. Playing nurse's aide repeatedly throughout the day and evening conflicted with my home preparations and came much too late to be beneficial.

In only a few days, my son Steve and I transformed our non-accessible home by adding ramps, chairlift, and duplicate wheelchair and commode on the second floor. Steve took charge of the physical logistics and conversion, first fumigating, then scrubbing and rearranging his old bedroom to accommodate the hospital bed. Next he moved furniture, pulled doors off hinges, and laid down sheets of plastic so that Herb might wheel his chair from kitchen and dining room to living room and back. He carried his father's desk and computer up from our basement office and rearranged the living room so that Herb might eventually feel inclined to use the word processor and Internet resources. And finally, he huddled with our health-care equipment provider and designed a set of ramps so we might easily move the wheelchair from the garage up over a series of steps into our back foyer.

Adding to the pressures of transitions, toileting, and insulin/heparin injections came the just-in-time arrival of a faulty glucose monitor. As my feelings of inadequacy, frustration, and danger mounted, I found myself running repeatedly to the bathroom and retching.

My husband and I survived this twenty-four-hour furlough but with an unnecessary level of stress. To this day I shudder at the memory of the awful strain that adequate preparation could have lessened!

Lessons Learned

Hire a full-time nurse to help you over the first few hurdles.

Home adjustment is challenging, whether your stroke survivor is fully or partially disabled, particularly if as caregiver you must administer complicated medications and injections. If you feel you are inadequately trained, ask others to help you. Under the best of circumstances, the overall situation is stressful and dangerous because of unfamiliar responsibilities, hazardous falls, and potential errors in drug administration.

Consider duplicate equipment.

Lugging a wheelchair and commode continually up a flight of stairs to a second level can easily and quickly wear out the caregiver. If you have a two-story home, arrange duplicate equipment (new or used) to ease the adjustment and strain. There are community organizations that can provide donated equipment at no cost.

Learn to operate medical devices before you go home.

Under Medicare regulations, durable medical equipment and instrumentation ordered by the hospital for the stroke survivor does not arrive until the day of discharge. This regulation leaves little time to learn new usage, programming, and applications. If your patient requires blood pressure and glucose monitoring, learn how to program and use these specific devices comfortably in the hospital before your patient comes home.

Purchase pill organizers.

Stroke survivors generally take a variety of medications throughout the day. From your local pharmacy, purchase a set of plastic pill organizers that sequentially divide the days of the week into segments. The organizer allows the caregiver to prepare several weeks of medications in advance while helping to prevent serious omissions and duplications.

Be patient with yourself.

The caregiver faces an abrupt change, one for which few of us are prepared. Above all, put safety first and then chart manageable expectations for yourself and your stroke survivor.

Consider a baby monitor.

Assuming the patient and caregiver sleep in separate rooms, this device relays all sounds.

Chapter 5

First Month at Home

Sometimes Good People with the Best of Intentions Can Make a Bad Situation Even Worse

The most physically challenging of all my new caregiver responsibilities was mastering the wheelchair. Lifting Herb's wheelchair and positioning it in the trunk of the car remained a huge problem. Custom-designed for left-handed control, it weighs approximately 55 pounds. The sequenced task involved collapsing the chair (which didn't collapse easily), separating the footrests and cushion, removing the tension rod (which required me to flip the chair over and get down on my hands and knees), and then loading it from the ground into the trunk. I had to remember to bend my knees to avoid back strain each time I lifted the chair to and from the trunk. Mastery of this task would give us independence and the ability to go to medical appointments and outside therapies.

I chose to use a home-nursing service for the first month, in the belief that I would have continuing support while Herb and I adjusted to the chair and our new status. I was wrong. The nurse, therapists, and bath person came in and out, often on their own schedules. This lack of control, exacerbated by my husband's secondary medical problems and frequent medical appointments, increased my overall stress level.

After hours, we followed homework sheets assigned by in-hospital and home therapists. One way or the other, Herb had to begin coordinating his body with the one-sided pyramid walker. And I had to hold his gait belt, learn to balance his new walking pattern, and catch any missteps.

After injections, bathing was the most frightening aspect of my new role as a caregiver. The wheelchair didn't fit through the bathroom door, the bench over the bathtub rocked unsteadily, and the shower water flooded the floor and walls. There was no way I was going to give my husband his first showers by myself. Instead, I stalled by giving him sponge baths until I could hire skilled support.

During our first month at home, we had two emergency runs, including a two-night hospital stay. Herb had already spent a total of almost eight weeks in the hospitals. He was covered by Medicare and an AARP supplement, and it was crucial that I understood our policies and whether these new expenses were still covered. Although I sometimes found myself in lengthy telephone queues, I had positive support from both groups as I explored the parameters of his insurance policies. People in these departments can be helpful!

Lessons Learned

Review your health insurance coverage as soon as possible.

Your policy should include catastrophic medical coverage. Recognize the parameters of your policy (or policies), particularly sections that deal with number of hospital days per incident, durable medical equipment, and therapies. Talk with a company representative to clarify any questions.

Consider a lightweight transit chair for travel.

The transit chair has less than half the poundage of a regular wheelchair, folds and lifts easily, and can remain in the car trunk. Look for a slightly used chair, which can be obtained at a substantial savings.

It is ideal for appointments, assuming you prefer, as I do, not to rely on availability of wheelchairs in medical facilities. If you are unable to boost this limited weight, a van and wheelchair lift become your best option.

Purchase durable clothing.

A moderately or fully handicapped stroke survivor has basic clothing needs – primarily garments that are absorbent, easy to put on, and durable enough to withstand repeated washing. Fleece pants with stretchable waistbands are ideal and adapt easily to long periods of sitting in a wheelchair. Look for loose clothing with zippered fronts for men. If you can sew, a Velcro opening is ideal.

Take home the hospital urinals.

You can't have too many plastic urinals. Collect as many as you can of your stroke survivor's urinals, which hospitals otherwise discard weekly and upon discharge. You can easily disinfect and refresh them with a solution of equal amounts bleach and water. If your male stroke survivor is unable to use the toilet, place urinals in convenient areas around your home. You can also purchase more urinals through a medical-supply business. A few sheets of toilet paper will catch the extra dripping.

Buy a backpack.

Choose one with three zippered compartments, particularly one with space for urinal, wipes, extra toilet paper, and plastic gloves (to be used by the caregiver).

Schedule daily caregiver exercise time and follow it.

Repeated bending and lifting can strain your back and muscles. Even in the midst of frantic, nonstop caregiver activity, build in time and space for stretching and exercise to strengthen and relax your body. In addition, squirrel away a few personal minutes daily to use in whatever way you find relaxing and reenergizing.

Recognize the limitations of agency home care.

Medicare-provided home care offers only minimal drop-in support and little overall coverage. The biggest advantage your transition month may give you is the time to regain limited energy before beginning out-patient rehab.

Begin outpatient rehab as soon as possible.

Every day counts in revitalizing muscles and limbs. In retrospect, I believe we should have skipped home nursing and begun the outpatient program sooner.

Enlist the help of family and friends.

You can't do everything on your own, especially at the beginning. If friends aren't available, seek out a volunteer group that provides such help, perhaps through your municipality, county, church, or synagogue. You'll need help to pick up medications, prepare healthy meals, or even cover for you as you step away for a few minutes.

Place a big calendar in a prominent place.

Buy one that has the full month at a glance and daily segments large enough to list multiple activities, then keep it where you will see it often during the day. It will help you organize and limit your activities and responsibilities. One rule of thumb: If you can't fit it all into the box or in the message reminders, you may have scheduled too many activities.

Try applesauce.

When your patient has difficulty swallowing and requires many pills in different sizes and shapes, try mixing a few pills at a time into a teaspoon of applesauce. As Mary Poppins advises, it helps the medicine go down.

Purchase a body wash that doesn't require rinsing.

This product permits easy sponging and allows your patient to go several weeks without a full shower or bath. I wish I had known about no-rinse wash during the first month.

Chapter 6
Transitioning to Our New Life
Ties That Bind and Support

Life became much harder after our son Steve left to resume the life that he'd placed on hold for three months. Before leaving, he insisted that I hire outside support, preferably young, attractive, and dynamic individuals, to come to our home and exercise his father several times daily. "Don't slacken the routine and don't worry about the cost," he said repeatedly. "Spend the money." If Herb had only a limited window of time in which to improve, Steve wanted us to make as great an effort as possible.

He was also concerned about the physical and emotional toll on me from stress, disruption, and continuing caregiver demands. "Use that time," he urged, "to give some thought to yourself and your future." Caught up in the urgency of Herb's situation, I tucked away his advice and, with all my power and strength of purpose, pushed my husband forward, taking intermittent but never long breaks. Within a few weeks, fatigue, stress, and the 24/7 routine caught up with me, and I knew it was time to get outside help.

Bringing in others to exercise and bathe Herb was a start. But I also needed a few hours away, knowing that my husband was in good hands. Through referrals and friends, a "home team" came together. The physical therapist at our new outpatient facility trained members of our team in transitions, gait-walking, and bed/chair exercises.

Even with a break of several hours twice a week, the pressure was still intense. I worried mostly about possible falls associated with toileting. The first fall came when Herb tried to lift himself to a sitting position at the edge of the bed to use the plastic urinal. Although the hosptal bed had safety guards on both sides, Herb was back in our own king-size bed and lacked that protection. I tried tucking the sheeting tightly under the mattress to secure him in place, but he pulled it out. In the middle of the night, I heard a thump. There he was, splayed on the floor. Fortunately, Steve had built a bench with a side handle that Herb could grab with his working left hand while I struggled to lift him. From this in-between level, he then used his pyramid walker to push up to a standing position while I pulled. The bench would continue to come in handy at various times.

Many friends wanted to visit in the first few months, but with only a few exceptions I discouraged them. While others might enjoy socializing, I found these visits difficult to fit into limited time along with the many complications I was managing.

Lessons Learned

Planning routine respite care is essential.

Fatigue makes caregivers grumpy. It can also lower resistance and make you ill. Make time to rest during the day and at night. You can't problem-solve and keep things in perspective when you are tired and feel backed into a corner. Ask friends for names of qualified caregivers. Recommendations from friends are more credible than referrals from agencies or a blind ad in the newspaper. Above all, check multiple references carefully.

Train people whom you already know and trust.

Seek people who are bright, enthusiastic, and strong enough to handle the moving and pivoting required by a partially or fully disabled survivor. Ask your outpatient physical therapist to train your team in proper gait techniques and exercises.

Establish a schedule.

Consistency and regularity help you gain better control of a difficult situation. Few days at the beginning will go the way you've planned, but a format helps both caregiver and survivor to adapt more easily to the routine and home life.

Discourage casual drop-in visitors.

At the beginning, the caregiver has a hectic pace, which is best maintained without the distraction of unscheduled company. Caregivers as well as survivors need downtime and a few treasured corners for retreat, without demands or interruptions, especially in the early weeks.

Join a caregiver support group.

Spend time with others in similar situations. Contact the social worker at your hospital to find out about groups that meet in your area. Some of these groups also have a simultaneous but separate group meeting for stroke survivors.

Prepare for falls.

Poor balance leads to falls. Few people have the strength to lift a partially paralyzed stroke survivor. Plan in advance. Consider a low bench with a handle positioned on the working side as an in-between step to help you maneuver your patient back into bed or wheelchair. It may take time but it is preferable to calling EMS.

Chapter 7

Medical Complications

When You Think Things Can't Get Any Worse, They Do

The statistics for stroke survivors are sobering. Of an estimated 700,000 Americans who have a first stroke, 5 to 14 percent will have another within one year. Even worse, 24 percent of women and 42 percent of men will have a second stroke within the first five years. Adding to the pressure, the risk for my husband (a man with preexisting diabetes) was two and a half times higher than for non-diabetic survivors.

To minimize his risk of another stroke, I focused on improving his eating and exercising patterns, and actively identifying medical problems before they became emergencies. An increasing series of secondary complications ratcheted up the continuing pressure. We experienced a wide range of problems from constipation, retention of urine and urinary-tract infections, and depression to sleep apnea and chronic facial pain. Along the way a previously missed cardiac condition and a pharmaceutical side effect that caused acute glaucoma also demanded attention.

Each problem generated more specialists and more appointments. Sometimes treatment for one problem led to a series of other steps. For example, a very strong antibiotic prescribed to combat Herb's urinary infection required frequent monitoring with blood tests, urine specimens, and follow-up appointments. A further diagnosis of iron-deficiency anemia required transfusions, thirteen weekly injections of iron, and repeated lab analysis. Because each problem was treated separately, we had as many as twenty specialists at one time.

Uneasy about a cardiac diagnosis, we traveled to another medi center for a second opinion from a board-certified cardiologist. SF advised me to identify a local medical manager able to coordinate Herb's medical treatment and be available to us during our frequent emergencies. Our new internist, who was not subject to frequent out-of-the-continent assignments like the first, agreed to respond to e-mails particularly when I had serious but non-emergency needs.

I also learned to organize copies of medical and pharmaceutical records in a medical loose-leaf folder, divided by medical specialties, in an effort to make sure the different specialists were aware of Herb's problems and could recognize any pharmaceutical conflicts and adjust medications as necessary.

Before each medical visit, I still prepare a one-page summary bulleting problems, new developments, questions, and a list of current medications with corresponding dosages and corresponding times when the medications are dispensed. A word processor allows me to update and revise the lists easily. These sheets are invaluable for me and our physicians.

Lessons Learned

Choose your physicians carefully.

Everyone needs an internist or primary care physician even without an emergency. Choose your physicians with care. Research (you may even "Google" on the Internet) your doctors and their history, how they practice, and whether they have any malpractice suits pending.

ook for training (board certification is a plus), referral by physicians whom you trust, willingness to manage your case, and an ability to communicate well. Find out how to alert your doctors when you spot a serious problem and require prompt response. Then put them through the test: If your physician is too busy to listen to your problems (be concise and prioritize the most severe first!), find one who will. Ask your doctor to review all your medications for problem interactions and continuing relevance.

Insist that your physicians speak understandable English.

Physician-speak is a language that lay people do not understand. As patients, we find medical terms far beyond our capabilities and training. While many courts provide translators for the adjudicated, medical systems do not. Insist that your physicians answer your questions and provide descriptions and instructions in everyday, understandable language. Raise questions and concerns. If you don't understand an instruction or explanation, ask again. You have a right to know. Conversely, if your first language is not English and you have problems understanding what your doctor is saying (or your doctor has problems understanding you), bring a translator with you so that there will be no misunderstandings on either side about this important information.

Recognize that stroke can precipitate many other conditions.

Often you may feel confused by many interlocking medical problems, each one treated in isolation. Question your rehab specialist or internist about a possible interaction between stroke and complications manifested by your survivor. You shouldn't have to figure this out on your own. Recovery takes time.

Research stroke complications.

Many of the complications affecting your stroke survivor may result from the overall brain injury. Although you may require several specialists, insist that your internist coordinate this treatment. Integrated teamwork, still unknown in many tertiary-care facilities, is a very effective approach because it treats the entire patient rather than isolated parts. Pain, just one possible complication, affects 5 percent of stroke survivors and often occurs at the time of stroke or even a year later.

Research stroke complications on your own using the Internet, available in most libraries, and a search engine such as Google. Identify medical websites that discuss stroke complications, using key words: stroke complications, stroke, and stroke rehabilitation. Your survivor may have one or more of these problems, or none, but at least you will know how to track and respond should any develop.

Consult with another specialist, preferably one outside your medical system.

Should you question specific aspects of the survivor's medical condition, treatment, or surgical recommendations, consult with a qualified specialist, preferably one who is board-certified and located in a system unrelated to your current hospital and physicians. Arrange for the transfer of pertinent records for review or carry them yourself – an excellent way to make sure they arrive on time. Most insurance plans cover a second opinion. In case of doubt, you should consider a third opinion.

Accept ultimate responsibility for managing your survivor's condition.

The caregiver or chosen advocate must take command. The doctor-patient relationship is not what it once was: Time slots are limited, appointments require long waiting periods, and overscheduled physicians have too little time to troubleshoot. Report unusual patterns and problems. Make your communications clear and concise.

Write down your questions and concerns before each medical appointment.

Time with your physician is limited. An appointment forces you to think through your priorities. Organize and write down questions, problems, and changes in medications in advance so that you allow more time for targeted discussion. Limit yourself to one side of one sheet of paper.

Participate in all decisions about your stroke survivor's treatment.

You and your physician should agree on exactly what will be done at each step of your survivor's care. Know who will be treating your patient, how long the treatment will last, and exactly what a new test or medication is likely to achieve.

Take notes and follow instructions.

Carry a pen and pad and write down all instructions and recommendations. If your doctor calls for significant changes, repeat them to ensure accuracy. If you have any question about instructions or find unexpected results or problems, contact your physician immediately.

Maintain your own medical records.

Request copies of reports from all specialists on your medical team. Assume that exchange among and within health-care institutions requires a long lag time. Your information will fill the gap. Keep a loose-leaf binder with separate sections for each medical problem. File and date copies of reports, discharge summaries, tests, and lists of medications in corresponding sections, beginning with the most recent report. Carry the binder with you when you travel, begin new therapy programs, or add new specialists to your medical roster.

Organize pharmaceutical records.

List each medication, dosage, quantity, time of day, and prescribing physician. Include over-the-counter products. A word processor will make it easier to store and update easily. Bring a current list to each medical and dental appointment (See *Appendix 5*).

Create a super-map for medications.

A medication map covers your entire day's scheduling. It plots when you give which medications, the dosage, and any other key information, including name of physician prescribing the medication and the date of the initial prescription. At one glance, the sheet will tell you what, when, and how much. Time slots on your map should correspond with those on your medicine pillbox (See *Appendix 3*).

Bring an updated list of medications to each medical and dental visit.

The realistic potential for side effects and drug interactions requires constant review. Know the medications your stroke survivor takes and why he/she takes them. Provide an updated list of medications and corresponding dosages at each appointment. Update all information regularly. A simple sheet of paper, preferably stored on a word processor, is much more efficient than trying to memorize complex names randomly or carrying bags of prescription bottles.

Arrange a separate place or box to store medications.

A self-contained plastic box is ideal. List by order of the day to correspond with your medication map. Also keep a pad where you store your medications so that you can write down any questions or problems for discussion at your next appointment.

Watch for harmful side effects.

Read pharmaceutical information on labels and enclosed instructions for usage directions and possible side effects (these instructions are called PPIs for Patient Prescription Information). Remain vigilant for symptoms associated with a new prescription. Some side effects that occur rarely may not be listed. Should something unusual but minor occur, monitor the problem and report to your physician. If the problem is acute, such as blurry vision, contact your ophthalmologist and/or internist immediately.

Chapter 8
Maneuvering through the Medical Maze
A Crash Course in Working through a Medical Bureaucracy

Medical institutions are huge bureaucracies. Fortunately, Herb has a well-qualified and responsive medical team, but assembling it was not easy. Our team crisscrosses two states and four hospital systems. For two troubling years, we found ourselves waiting as long as three hours in the waiting rooms of most specialists and were unable to bundle appointments. The lack of medical integration was even more worrisome.

Because of Herb's many secondary complications, we had about twenty specialists at any one time. Each appointment, preceded by frantic searches in the parking garage to find a handicapped parking spot wide enough to move Herb to his wheelchair, required runs through long hospital corridors. In the first three years, I had few opportunities to bundle appointments and tests on the same day or, even better, the same part of the day.

Each specialist, even those within the same system, worked in a vacuum, oblivious to Herb's other medical problems. Few exchanged information or reviewed records with others on our roster. I kept asking: Why won't they share records and treat the patient rather than individual parts? Who puts it all together?

After many upsetting nights, I awoke with the solution. Herb and I were professional communicators, paid to sort through disparate elements to identify and communicate their strategic common denominator. Why couldn't I just apply our skills to this situation?

I faxed a memo to each of our specialists, identifying everyone on Herb's medical team by name, specialty, and telephone and fax numbers. The memo summarized significant developments that had occurred over the previous two weeks, listed current medications, and introduced Herb's new internist-case manager. I explicitly stated that all future reports must be sent to our internist and cardiologist with a copy to me. No exceptions (See *Appendix 6*).

The system worked, not perfectly but well. To help the process, we compiled the records in our three-ring medical binder and carried them with us, particularly to new appointments. Those specialists who didn't cooperate were replaced.

Lessons Learned

Coordinate diverse specialists.

Cooperation with your internist/case manager and diverse team, especially in a complicated case, is vital. You may have to initiate this communication by providing a composite list of all your specialists' names and addresses. Should you feel that a specialist does not exchange pertinent information in a timely and helpful manner or that your request is treated brusquely, replace the uncooperative physician with one who will work with you. (See *Appendix 4* for a sample summary sheet.)

Recognize your responsibility to share timely information.

The patient's advocate has a responsibility to share information, arrive on time for appointments, and bring questions, observations, and updated records from outside consults. However, be judicious and work through your questions and problems in advance so that you do not take advantage of the physician's time.

Follow treatment directions.

You have a responsibility to follow treatment directions. Write these down during the medical appointment. Arrange follow-up appointments on a regular basis. Request extra appointments only when absolutely urgent. Also check whether your internist and/or rehab specialist accepts e-mail as a means for communicating perplexing questions. Although it may lack the immediacy of a telephone call, the Internet promotes an exchange of communications while minimizing unnecessary medical appointments and telephone calls.

Bundle appointments.

It is fatiguing for patient and caregiver, especially one with a walker or wheelchair, to be forced repeatedly into a series of separate appointments on separate days within the same complex. Ask the appointment scheduler to bundle two or more appointments on the same day. If your request is denied, appeal to a supervisor.

Organize and maintain a list of your physicians' business cards.

Organized information is vital in an emergency. Request business cards from each doctor and anyone on the doctor's staff you might need to speak with, and store them alphabetically in a special business card file. The plastic sleeves allow flexibility for rearranging information. As an alternative, wrap a rubber band around the pile of cards. Each card should include printed name, address, medical specialty, telephone and fax numbers, and an optional e-mail address. For fast, easy reference, list your patient's hospital identification number and copies of insurance and supplementary insurance cards in the top sleeve of the organizer.

Break through the telephone logjam when you have a serious medical need.

Medical offices are notorious for long telephone waits. Jump in and say "No" when the secretary asks whether she can put you on hold. State your serious need and ask for immediate help at the beginning of your phone comments. Otherwise, yours will not stand out from all the many calls in the office queue.

You can appeal poor or indifferent treatment.

Assuming that you have unsuccessfully tried all available means to contact your physician with legitimate concerns, to organize appointments, or request copies of medical records, several options remain open. First, request help from your hospital's ombudsman. Next, contact your hospital system's chief executive officer (through the main number). The person who takes your call can usually direct you to the proper channel for resolution. If you are still unsuccessful – assuming that you have a choice – switch to another health-care system.

Chapter 9
Caregiver's Anger
"Anger Management" Is an Oxymoron

My anger was across the board. I was angry at our medical institution for allowing "a small stroke in a prime area of real estate" to become a massive wipeout. I was angry at the understaffed emergency room. I was angry at the hospital staff who failed to identify Herb's rapid deterioration as he lay hooked to sophisticated monitors in the neurological unit. I was angry at inept and indifferent nursing. And I was deeply angry about Herb's casual acceptance of diabetes and the corresponding risks that I believed led to the stroke.

At the bottom of all the anger, I blamed Herb for getting us into this situation. I deeply resented his refusal now to help himself. But maybe I was angriest with myself for not demanding a logical reason from our medical institution for the persistent pain in Herb's left arm three years before the stroke. I felt guilty that I had not sought an outside consult much earlier.

My life had now become a nonstop race from one hospital and therapy program to another. I desperately missed our former life. We had shared a successful consulting business with many international trips.

Pulling away from family and friends, I made fewer phone calls and felt little incentive to make it through the day. Sometimes I wondered whether this empty shell of husband and life was all I would have in the future. I cried often from loneliness, frustration, fear, and exhaustion.

Our psychologist saw that I was fraying and discussed caregiver wear-out and illness. She repeatedly advised me to hire a permanent caregiver and arrange more personal time to pursue my own interests. My cardiologist strongly recommended that for my health I carve out at least two one-week trips a year by myself. How, I asked, could I take on more expense when we were already paying many hundreds of dollars a month for at-home support and therapies?

Both suggestions made more sense as I came to realize that enforced togetherness creates friction points and leads to burnout. Both Herb and I benefit from the limited time away from one another, and I return refreshed and ready to pick up the mantle once again.

Lessons Learned

Caregiver time-out is mandatory.

For both you and your stroke survivor, burnout is unaffordable. Time off from a 24/7 working schedule is imperative. A caregiver must break away once in a while for longer periods of even a week or two to come up for air.

Choose your battles.

Personal grievances create unnecessary baggage. Differentiate big problems from small nuisances and address only those problems that directly affect your stroke survivor's recovery.

Set priorities.

When caregivers get very busy and short of time, self-care comes last. Thoughtless eating and skipping meals, skimping on exercise, getting too little sleep, and failing to allow for some downtime can take the biggest toll of all on your immune system. Put yourself first, because if you get sick, both you and your stroke survivor go down.

Share your feelings and find ways to vent your anger.

Sort through your feelings with a trusted friend, preferably another caregiver. You may feel guilty, thinking you should have recognized and done more to correct bad habits or symptoms that led to the stroke. You may also feel depressed and frightened about losing your loved one. It helps to talk out these emotions so they don't fester. Consider professional help if you are deeply depressed or feel frustrated confiding to friends not in a similar situation.

Ask for help.

Assume that people – even willing friends – don't know much about strokes. Share your needs, even when all you want is a hug, a few words of encouragement, or a drink with a friend. Accept help, but be specific: a dog walked, a cup of coffee, respite care for a half-hour. The window of opportunity closes after the first few months and most people will stop asking.

Don't negate your own existence.

Serving as caregiver does not make you less of a person. As a human being you have value and needs in your own right. Although you are harried, pushed, and stressed, find whatever it is that helps you relax and recharge. Specifically create space for yourself, your personal care, meals, and pursuits you find relaxing. These can coincide with nap times, but you may also choose to stretch your day by rising earlier or going to bed later than your spouse.

Cut as many corners as you possibly can.

Be realistic: You don't have to choose the hardest way each time. Other people will assume that you can do it all, but you know you can't... and you don't want to. Concentrate on your stroke survivor, your immediate family members, and yourself, and feel free to reject other responsibilities.

Forget about guilt.

Guilt consumes more energy than caregiving and is a luxury you can't afford. You will make mistakes. We all do. Divide your world into life-and-death situations and choose life. Don't sweat the rest.

Chapter 10
The Outpatient Therapy Program
Centimeter by Centimeter, We Inch Our Way Forward

Therapists with their unflagging "can do" spirit are the heroes and heroines of our story. Herb was not an exercise enthusiast before his stroke, and this omission, combined with a preexisting neuromuscular disease, complicates his current efforts to walk. Our children once characterized their father as "the kind of athlete who puts on sunglasses and drives through a park on a Sunday."

Outpatient rehabilitation at the first center lasted for almost a year. All three therapies, including physical, occupational, and speech, met three times each week in consecutive one-hour sessions built around a one-hour break for lunch and rest. Since the center was a half-hour from our home, it made sense to bundle these appointments. His rehab physician, also at the same location, remained a vital part of the team for the first two years and continued to extend the program as long as Herb met his goals. At the beginning, Herb couldn't square his shoulders or take more than a couple of steps with his pyramid walker, but he worked hard and steadily improved.

Under Medicare rules, the nasty word in rehab therapy is "plateau," loosely defined by others who came before us as a failure to make progress. A physician must recommend and provide a written prescription to initiate therapy. The stated period usually covers a dozen or more sessions. However, the program is renewable, provided that the patient advances within stated government guidelines. But, should that patient simply lock in at any level (hence plateau), the therapy program stops.

Herb's speech therapist at the outpatient rehab center deserves the greatest credit for his recovery. At the beginning, as he was feeling humbled and useless, she and Herb discussed his career prior to the stroke, along with his frustrating inability now to exchange words and thoughts. Kathy recognized Herb's capabilities and by building on his interests helped him reestablish the connections. Herb's cognitive functioning, although somewhat disjointed by illness, seemed otherwise intact. Rather than concentrate only on improving his slurred speech, she tailored a therapy program specifically for him that focused on language expression, word retrieval, and organizing thoughts. Her exercises guided Herb back to his word processor. Later, she worked on sequencing events, logical thinking, and writing progression. Within months, Herb became more facile with the keyboard and learned to punctuate as well as shift between upper and lower cases.

After completing the first outpatient program, we advanced to a second therapy center only minutes from our home. Armed with a new Medicare-approved prescription, this time written by our internist, Herb attended therapy there twice a week for another year. He learned to do deep knee bends in the water on his weakened right leg and use an underwater treadmill to rebuild the muscles of his lower right leg and thigh. His therapists stressed that contact therapy time alone is insufficient to reach desired goals and requires daily at-home reinforcement.

Herb's occupational therapist insisted that Herb learn to dress himself and suggested various devices that might assist him. The first time Herb dressed himself the task took more than an hour, and when he finished he was drenched in perspiration. He subsequently reduced the task to ten minutes.

Formal therapies concluded just before our second-year marker and Herb graduated with honors. He had reached most of the goals set by his therapists.

We continue to seek as much physical therapy as possible. With a private membership at the aquatics center, we independently use their special fitness equipment. Herb's physical therapist trained me to operate the varied Nautilus equipment and provide basic training. We try to work out at least two times a week. In addition, in conjunction with several pilot fitness programs, we have a treadmill in our home that Herb uses another three times each week.

Sustained therapeutic practices keep Herb from being imprisoned in a nursing home. At the same time, he must exert great effort to maintain his current level and even more to advance. To act otherwise will mean regression.

Herb's ultrasounds demonstrate a very positive outgrowth of his exercise program: increasing blood flow to constricted parts of his brain.

Lessons Learned

Identify knowledgeable and caring therapists.

Search for therapists and programs willing to tap into the stroke survivor's interests; these can be powerful motivators. Talk with therapists about what constitutes reasonable goals and expectations, and make sure you concur.

Supplement formal therapy programs.

Recovery requires tremendous reinforcement. Home practice must become part of the daily routine. Most therapists provide lots of homework. Use those materials to develop a daily program for pre-scribed therapies, and create a similar program for continued practice after formal therapy concludes.

Get around the dreaded "plateau."

Medicare and other insurance programs require that the stroke survivor make steady progress. Ask your therapist to explain these guidelines. As one program ends, find another with a different emphasis and request a new medical authorization.

Train your survivor to use a word processor.

Stroke survivors who have difficulty expressing their thoughts verbally may discover that a word processor is an effective communications outlet. Special keyboards designed for one-handed use may facilitate the activity. Some systems also use speech synthesis and recognition for those with little movement or voice.

Continue exercise after therapy programs conclude.

Don't slacken your efforts even after your survivor graduates from ther-apies. Find other programs and centers on your own, and continue to progress.

Search for experimental programs.

The National Institutes of Health, Veterans Administration, and Claude D. Pepper Legacy programs are among a number now researching the effects of stroke and searching for methods to aid improvement.

Ask your rehab physician, research the Internet and your library, and read stroke publications. These programs hold promise and do not limit post-stroke achievements by timetable.

Learn when to step back and let your stroke survivor take over.

You can't and don't want to do everything. Gradually allow benign neglect to become the order of the day. Sometimes building independence is painful.

Chapter 11

Friends and Family

Finding Support When Your Back Is Against the Wall

Stroke is a life-changing experience. Nothing is as it was before. Outsiders who contribute warmth and support are welcome; those who draw energy away are not.

Our family, friends, and neighbors continue to provide immeasurable support. Many have hovered about us from the beginning. Others disappeared after sending the token card or gift. Perhaps they worried Herb's stroke might be contagious. Or maybe they felt uncomfortable trying to hold a conversation with him.

No doubt I antagonized some people by not taking phone calls at the beginning when everything was so frantic. Special, well-tested friends and family members continued despite my rebuffs. I talked with immediate family members by cell phone early in the morning and late at night while I walked the dog. Time restrictions likewise limited e-mail, but with a few extra clicks one message could reach many.

The warm neighbors and sense of community reinforce our decision to remain in our home rather than shift to a more accessible condo elsewhere. Neighbors offer comfort and support in many different ways. A number have stepped forward to run errands, walk the dog, visit Herb, and share periodic dinners and desserts. During the blackout of August 2003, when most of the eastern United States and parts of Canada lost power and water, neighbors knocked on our door to check in and offer help. Some dropped off cases of bottled water. Others have told us to call them in an emergency, day or night. In our former lives, Herb and I often reached out to help others in need. Now we are recipients. We try hard to express our appreciation.

Even now we encourage our visitors to speak slowly and allow Herb time to respond. We find small groups more conducive to an exchange than larger ones. And as a caregiver, I find I must discipline myself not to cut Herb off by jumping to conclusions.

Family, friends, and neighbors have paved the way for Herb's reentry into the world with patience, understanding, and thoughtfulness. It takes the good nature of others to encourage you to move out once again into the larger community.

Lessons Learned

Don't isolate yourselves.

Friends and neighbors may feel awkward and not know exactly what to say or do, but they still want to visit. Arrange a short block of time for them to say hello. Don't worry about serving food. Also provide a departure signal, such as when you stand up, nod your head, or point to the door.

Establish ground rules.

People don't know what to say or do in the face of serious illness. Set up a few ground rules and explain them in advance. If the stroke survivor has difficulty speaking or following a conversation, suggest that only one person speak at a time, speaking slowly and allowing time for response, whether it be in words, a grunt, or a nod. For the patient, crowds are overwhelming and lead to discouragement.

Consider stroke clubs.

Seek new friends who share understanding and compassion with both caregiver and survivor. Many of the programs are informative and helpful. You'll meet people who understand your situation and can provide advice for particular needs and concerns.

Entertain over dessert and coffee.

Later in the recovery, as you feel more confident, arrange small gatherings under controlled circumstances. Make it casual and easy. Even consider disposable dishes. Empower your guests to bring the food if they insist.

Meet friends at restaurants.

Get around the hassles of difficult logistics by meeting in an accessible restaurant that you have scouted in advance. An outing offers a nice change of pace and avoids the awkwardness and fear of trying to manage at inaccessible homes.

Chapter 12
Food-Smart Recovery

If It Has No Salt, Fat, or Sugar, It Probably Has No Taste … But So What?

Learning to practice smart eating was a critical step in Herb's recovery. His entrenched eating patterns simply had to change. Diabetes is bad enough, but discovering that high blood sugar can bring on another stroke caused me to draw a line in Herb's mashed potatoes and make diet a cornerstone of our recovery program.

I went ballistic trying to follow all possible rules to bring down his high sugar and cholesterol levels. I bought many of the trendy books but was surprised to find that low fat did not necessarily equate with low sugar. The upshot was that Herb, an emaciated 143 pounds on his return home, stopped eating and said he preferred to go hungry. He had no appetite. Nor did I. The food I so painstakingly researched, shopped for, and prepared turned us both off. Meanwhile Herb's hematocrit level dropped precipitously and he had critical iron-deficiency anemia. Our internist attributed the cause to chronic illness and related complications. I disagreed and discovered that lean, red meat had a positive effect in raising his hematocrit level.

Out went the books and the nutritionist. Back came eggs, French toast, and pancakes made with egg whites – along with limited, low-calorie syrup. Lots of vegetables make up our diet today, but we focus on the ones that Herb has always enjoyed: carrots, string beans, spinach, yams, and potatoes. We use prodigious amounts of dried lentils, split peas, and lima beans. Sometimes unfamiliar dark greens and root vegetables creep into his soups but are readily camouflaged by the food processor.

My reward comes in plotting Herb's glucose levels, now usually within normal ranges albeit with oral medications. His quarterly hemoglobin HBA1C-glucose rating remains at under 6, another significant measurement of our success.

Ever-changing food controversies continue to confuse me. Too much salt versus too little, fish high in omega-3s versus mercury poisoning, red meat versus puffs of air are all issues without resolution. Rather than follow a changing food pyramid, I prefer to focus on common sense and tangible results.

After all my fruitless efforts to change our pattern of eating, I learned the most important lesson of all. One can win a Pyrrhic victory but lose the war. Unless my husband enjoys his food, preparations and substitutions are useless.

Lessons Learned

Talk to a nutritionist about your stroke survivor's specific food requirements.

The more you know, the more in control you are. Before making any dietary changes, either seek help from a nutritionist familiar with your medical needs or independently research the problems, foods, and ingredients to avoid. Learn about portion size and how to limit certain foods while emphasizing others.

Always read food labels.

Bring a magnifying glass when you shop. Even foods that seem similar can have very different nutritional values, sugar content, and calories.

Prepared foods, particularly the "low-carbohydrate" kind, generally include surprise ingredients, such as sodium and fats, to make them tasty.

Choose worthy substitutes.

Diet is a key element in controlling blood sugar and high cholesterol. Low-fat dessert novelties made with sugar substitutes offer good taste when used in moderation. New buttery spreads made from natural oils have no hydrated or trans fats. And ground buffalo offers a lean, tasty hamburger.

Seek foods that reduce high glucose and cholesterol levels.

Certain foods, such as dried beans, can actually bring down high glucose and cholesterol levels. Some fat is necessary for your diet, but choose "good" fat that is unsaturated. Adding just a little olive oil adds taste and eliminates "bad" cholesterol.

Don't forget the fiber.

Many highly processed foods have zero fiber, so necessary to regularity. Whole grains, fruits, beans, and other vegetables are high in fiber, which fights off bad cholesterol and minimizes chronic constipation.

Exercise common sense.

Common sense and compromise must coexist in modifying the stroke survivor's eating patterns and quality of life. Food should be appealing by eye and taste, whatever the dietary modifications. When food becomes boring or too regimented, it's just not worth eating.

Chapter 13
Toileting Nightmares
The World Is a Difficult Place,
and a Little Help Wouldn't Be So Terrible

How I wish that somewhere in all the medical discussions, the pages and pages of literature, and the conversations with other caregivers someone had talked to me about the ultimate in caregiver survival: DEPENDs, DEPENDs, DEPENDs.

Stroke attacks all bodily functions, but toileting is seldom discussed in lay terms. I learned only after great anguish that urinary frequency is a prevalent side effect. The toileting function became even more complex for us because Herb could not independently walk to the bathroom or use a plastic urinal. Our lives revolve around this now immortalized urinal. Five or six nest in prime locations around our home.

As we ventured out from our home to the wider world, I found myself frustrated by the lack of available facilities to accommodate my husband's needs. There was not a trip, visit, excursion, or walk where right in the middle of things – and usually at the most inconvenient spot with the least hygienic conditions imaginable -- he suddenly and absolutely had to go. Urgency is a fact of life.

Because Herb has little use of his right side, poor balance, and only one usable hand, he requires assistance to stand, sit, unzip, and wipe. At most, we have three minutes, usually fewer, to find a bathroom. Unisex facilities are not universal. Even in large medical complexes, we are challenged to find handicap-accessible toilets that accommodate both of us and the wheelchair in the same room.

According to federal guidelines, a handicap-accessible bathroom must have both door and stall wide enough to accommodate a wheelchair. In real life, these rules aren't enforced. Hospitals and medical office buildings are the most flagrant offenders, but the problem is widespread. The rare unisex/family/wheelchair-accessible toilets are often hidden at the end of long hallways and behind heavy doors. Most resemble broom closets and often double as storage areas with boxes of toilet paper, hand wipes, and other cleaning paraphernalia piled to the ceiling.

I spent months devising a way to keep Herb dry for several hours at a time when toilets and urinals weren't available. The urologist prescribed a variety of medications from Detrol LA to Flomax to lessen the urinary frequency, but we discontinued both because of dangerous side effects.

On our own, we tried Depends, the adult diaper. To include extra absorption, I inserted a feminine super-super napkin. I subsequently discovered an insert specifically tailored to adults. The combination works well, but the downside is a perceptible ammonia odor. Built-in protection has brought the outside world much closer and removed many prior constraints. And it has helped me to feel less stressed out! We can now sit through an entire movie or play, take drives in the country, and even participate in a lecture without panicking about when, where, or how quickly we must find relief.

Lessons Learned

DEPENDs, DEPENDs, DEPENDs.

Adult protection is a fact of life. With its use you can travel, attend exhibitions and performances, and not worry about "accidents." Don't leave home without it. Look for the ones with side tabs for easy application and removal even while fully dressed.

More reasons for a backpack.

Choose one with several zippered compartments. Carry a urinal, wipes, plastic gloves, and toilet seat covers along with a change of clothing, if necessary. The bag attaches easily to the back of a wheelchair.

Scout facilities in advance.

We now work harder to anticipate our needs in advance. Don't assume that restaurants, theaters, and museums address your needs automatically. Call ahead; visit the facilities; make your needs known.

Become an advocate.

Public indifference often stems from a lack of familiarity with specific needs of the disabled. Should you encounter situations in public areas that are not handicap-accessible, complain to the proper authorities and ask what corrections they plan to make.

Chapter 14
Travels with Herb
Discovering a Widening World

Today, international travel is beyond our reach. Long stretches spent sitting on airplanes threaten blood clots, narrow aisles are dangerous for a pyramid walker, and airplane toilets simply do not accommodate our needs. Even short hops don't seem worth the cost or the effort, especially when you factor in additional time for early arrivals, security checks, and transfers to a rental car while you're transporting wheelchair, walker, and suitcases.

It seems faster, easier, and generally more convenient just to drive. No longer spur-of-the-moment people, we plan our trips far ahead, particularly to reserve handicap-accessible hotel accommodations. Family homes are generally off-limits for overnight stays because of their steps, narrow bathrooms, and tight bedroom arrangements.

Hotels are also difficult. Although I expected stronger support through the Americans with Disabilities Act, I've come to realize its limitations. Seldom do we find wheelchair and toilet/shower accessibility. We've crossed many leading hotel chains off our list because of staff indifference and failure to process our handicap request.

Our specifications include a nonsmoking room, early check-in, portable high-rise commode fitted on top of the toilet seat, toilet bars, and roll-in shower. Even if we're assigned the correct room, which is rare, we must wait for a maintenance man to carry in and position the toilet seat extender and requisite attachments. Sometimes it still bears stains from the previous user. On other occasions we'll wait while yet another member of the housekeeping staff carries in a separate chair for the roll-in shower. We also require extra towels, especially to dry the bathroom floor after a shower and before Herb stands up. As another hassle, the order is not passed along to housekeeping, and we must make a new request daily.

With research and good luck we have identified kinder, gentler accommodations in cities we visit often. Pivoting around the proverbial one-tank gas trip, Herb and I seek wheelchair-conducive vacations that center on theaters, concerts, and university lectures. Like everything else in our lives, I'm learning to draw limits and not stretch beyond what I, as the caregiver, find easy and comfortable.

Lessons Learned

Make motel/hotel arrangements directly through in-house reservations.

The local hotel is usually more responsive to handicap requests than a central toll-free office that guarantees only a room and does not have specific room information to meet your needs. When you call, ask to speak with the in-house desk supervisor or manager. State your requirements (i.e., handicap-accessible, nonsmoking room with high-rise toilet seat and bars, roll-in shower, shower seat, and refrigerator) and specify if you want guaranteed early or late arrival. Request a formal acknowledgment by fax, e-mail, or letter confirming these details. It will come in handy on your arrival should you find certain arrangements lacking.

Exercise caution in accepting floor assignments.

If your stroke survivor is wheelchair-bound or on a walker, consider what might happen in the unlikely event of fire or other catastrophe when elevators are shut off and stairs offer the only accessible means of escape.

Request extra towels.

Towels keep the bathroom floor dry after a shower, especially when the floor lacks a central drain. Ask for double the number you require, and hide extras in a dresser drawer. That way, you won't have to wage the same fight daily.

Keep a travel file.

Keep a record of hotels with specific room numbers that have met your needs. This information will come in handy when you or someone you know makes a repeat visit. Request the room number directly through in-service registration.

Discuss special food restrictions with the restaurant chef.

If you have special dietary limitations and plan to take most of your meals at the same hotel or restaurant, it is helpful to work through dinner choices with the chef, preferably in advance.

Recognize your travel limitations.

Travel, whether by air or car, requires planning and arrangements, packing and unpacking, and lots of solo responsibility. Recognize your financial and energy limitations, and seek ways to ease the process.

Chapter 15
The Costs No One Talks About
Plan Ahead

When Herb and I planned for retirement, we did our best to project our future financial needs. In many respects, we were far off the mark. More than half our current expenditures never appeared on that list. We didn't factor in the cost of chronic and debilitating illness. Also absent was the long-term-care policy that I initiated for myself after Herb's stroke. We assumed our good health and business would continue indefinitely. Had our financial consultant suggested that we include an additional $40,000 to $50,000 per year for all the ongoing health-care expenses we now face, we both would have scoffed.

During the initial months when Herb was oblivious to the broader world, I couldn't ask him where he had filed certain information or, when I did find a file, how to process it. Fortunately, I was well aware of our finances and had knowledgeable professionals to turn to, specifically our broker and accountant, who provided vital counsel.

Herb's timing was fortunate. He was 66 when he had his stroke and already on Medicare. Had we *not* had an excellent supplemental policy, our savings would have evaporated rapidly. There would be no future earned income as I willingly became a full-time caregiver.

Medicare covered Herb's hospital and rehab expenses in full along with costly specialists, medical tests, surgeries, home health care, durable medical equipment, and extensive therapies. Medicare and the American Association of Retired Persons (AARP's J Program) have to this date not rationed care or denied even one legitimate expense.

In contrast to many less expensive health-care programs, we have flexibility to choose specialists and consultants in other health-care systems and states.

I use Quicken software, a valuable tool for categorizing and logging checks, credit-card receipts, and out-of-pocket cash expenses related to Herb's medical and home-adaptation needs. Our expenses accumulate quickly, especially for pharmaceuticals and home care. Organized and tabulated, they make up a substantial IRS deduction.

Lessons Learned

Plan ahead.

Stroke gives little warning. You don't want to find yourself searching for lost records in the midst of your sudden shock and loss.

Save as much as possible with the knowledge that rainy days do come. Long before illness strikes, choose your health and long-term insurance policies wisely. Make sure your finances, will, durable medical powers of attorney, and insurance policies are in order, with appropriate forms signed and notarized. Both spouses must know the amount of savings to draw upon and how to locate pertinent records and files, e.g., all bank accounts; mutual fund and brokerage holdings; safe-deposit box; vehicle titles; home mortgage; medical insurance; life insurance; Social Security benefits; retirement and annuity benefits; credit cards and traveler's checks; unpaid salary, IRAs, 401 (k), pension, and profit-sharing; workers' compensation benefits; and will. Discuss plans with your family lawyer, financial advisor, and accountant in advance.

Keep multiple copies of your durable medical power of attorney and living will on record.

Make sure critical information is clear and accessible to both partners before a medical catastrophe. Copies should be on file with your internist and hospital of choice as well as in your home records within easy reach. Keep one copy in the loose-leaf medical-records binder you've assembled.

Establish a formal power-of-attorney document.

This legal authority permits the operating spouse to sign legal documents, request medical information, and handle other formal transactions on behalf of the patient.

Keep accurate tax records.

Use accounting software and maintain accurate, up-to-date records. Hire an accountant who is well versed in such areas as health-care expenses and deductions.

Invest in long-term-care insurance for the caregiving spouse.

Whatever the other expenses, this one is basic and concerns your own future needs.

Monitor medical bills vigilantly.

Know your insurance coverage well, and take time to assess whether incoming bills are legitimate. Mistakes happen.

Don't pay rogue medical bills.

You are entitled to an itemized statement, even a daily one, if necessary. If the billing department does not correct bills that you can prove are in error, contact the hospital's financial ombudsman. Request the representative's name and a written record of the correction. Keep track of each person to whom you've spoken. Use a full sheet of paper and list date, name, and related comments.

Disregard mounting financial statements and pressures while your bill is in dispute. As a last resort, write to the chief executive of the medical facility giving you grief. Many companies now have specialized customer-service SWAT teams that field comments directed to that office. Rest assured that your complaint is not their only one.

Chapter 16

Harnessing Pharmaceutical Costs

Stretching Medications and Limited Dollars: Pharmaceuticals, a Huge Drain

Herb required twenty medications daily at an average monthly cost of almost $1,500 for the first two post-stroke years. With prenegotiated AARP prices, it seemed to make little difference where we filled our prescriptions. For convenience, I chose a local pharmacy. The downside was that Herb quickly exceeded his plan's $3,000 reimbursement maximum within the first six months of each year. We were on our own, albeit at an agreed-upon rate, for the remaining period. The time came to seek cost-saving initiatives and stretch his maximum to cover as much of the year as possible.

Lessons Learned

Discuss pharmaceutical needs with your physicians.

Enlist their support to prescribe quarterly prescriptions that you can purchase in bulk. Bulk purchase usually saves money but, before you order, first check for adverse side effects and whether you will require that prescription for the full period.

Comparison-shop for your pharmaceuticals.

Check all prices carefully and consider the steps toward cost savings that follow.

Use generics or lower-priced alternatives whenever possible.

Physicians often prescribe the newest and often most expensive medications when a generic drug will do the same job. Ask both your physician and pharmacist about workable substitutes. Generics are less expensive, particularly at some national chains and local discount pharmacies, which accept AARP's negotiated prices. One large warehouse chain, Costco, lists pharmaceutical prices on the Internet for ease of comparison.

Split pills.

Purchase and halve double-dose tablets for greater value since many drugs cost the same regardless of dosage. A $5 pill-splitter easily and accurately cuts most tablets.

Consider Canadian pharmacies.

With mostly nongeneric "designer" pharmaceuticals on Herb's list, my next step was to purchase prescriptions directly from Canada. After researching articles, online price comparisons, and personal recommendations, I chose a Canadian pharmacy that maintains our faxed prescription lists, ordered in quarterly refill quantities. I call its toll-free phone number, fax in new prescriptions, and charge the bundled reorder to my credit card. New prescriptions generally require three weeks, and renewals take two weeks or less. AARP reimburses one-half the cost of the three-month supply. There is currently no delivery charge. The savings are sometimes as high as 50 percent per order over local and chain pharmacies. Canadian prescription costs have increased with the decline in value of the U.S. dollar and as pharmaceutical manufacturers attempt to limit Canadian exports. Costs of medications in our local pharmacies are rising even faster. It remains to be seen whether Medicare pharmaceutical plans will actually prove more economical and as unrestrictive as purchases from Canadian pharmacies.

Buy in bulk.

You can find discounts when you purchase in bulk. Check the pricing and find the cost of each prescription by dividing number of pills into the total cost. Use this comparison analysis when evaluating possible benefits. But use this purchasing method only for standard pills that you feel confident you will use. Test a new drug by starting with the smallest possible quantity.

Request samples.

Pharmaceutical companies provide many samples to physicians. When starting on a new medication, we test it first in smaller quantity for adverse reactions rather than discard a three-month supply. In addition, I request samples of current prescriptions at the end of each appointment. Using samples can mean as many as three or four additional weeks in savings. Over the course of a year, these savings have sometimes added up to $1,000.

Prune the pharmaceuticals list.

We've had specialists whom we rarely see again prescribe medications. These prescriptions can easily continue into perpetuity. At each visit, we ask our internist and cardiologist to review our list of medications and recommend which, if any, we can remove.

Maintain contacts with local pharmacies.

Pharmaceuticals that have been on the market for a long time, such as Herb's long-acting nitroglycerin capsules, are often priced so low that large chains and Canadian pharmacies find little incentive to carry them. Local pharmacies oblige us with convenience, fast fulfillment, and accessibility. We turn to them when there isn't a huge price differential or with new prescriptions that must be filled immediately.

Donate unused or unfinished prescriptions.

Organizations in your area (such as free clinics) can benefit from prescriptions you've abandoned before their expiration dates. Your contribution may be a tax deduction.

Investigate patient-assistance programs.

Various drug companies offer special programs called patient-assistance programs (PAPs), which discount certain pharmaceuticals. Criteria vary with each company. Type the company name into Google or another search engine to find a direct link to the appropriate home page. (For more general information on PAPs, go to www.rxassist.org or www.needymeds.com/apps.taf.)

Medicare D.

Medicare D is another story; you'll need to do considerable research to determine whether the program offers you the best advantage for both your prescription needs and your finances.

Chapter 17

What Happens
When the Caregiver Gets Sick

When the Bough Breaks, the Cradle Will Fall

Early on a Sunday morning in our 32nd post-stroke month, I was awakened by a strange leg cramp. I roused myself and tried to walk it off, but as the day progressed, pain advanced down my leg. It became increasingly difficult to stand. I managed with Herb's chairlift and pyramid walker to carry up breakfast and lunch for him, and let the dog out for his breaks. But I was unable to reach our respite-care worker to ask for his help.

By dinnertime, I couldn't lift my leg and I became more frantic. Herb needed urinal-container changes and was beginning to grump at me because he hadn't eaten dinner. I felt isolated. Our closest neighbors were out of town. A snowstorm was raging with whiteout conditions and I hesitated to call others.

I managed to reach Otis, our respite-care worker, in the early evening, and he promised to come immediately and remain with Herb for however long it required. I finally was able to dial 911 and seek help for myself. The EMS team arrived within minutes. I grabbed my cell phone as they carried me out on a stretcher.

The entire experience shook me profoundly. Suddenly facing my own mortality was terrifying as I realized that my poor health or injury could easily destroy our fragile balance. Were I unable to care for us, we would have no other recourse than for both of us to go to an assisted-living or nursing facility. Other than Otis, I had no backup.

That next day, as I lay helpless and alone in the big hospital, it was up to me to notify our children and close family members, and tell them where I was.

Neighbors and friends later chastised me for not calling them day or night in an emergency. But just to be extra sure, I scheduled a home interview with a nursing service and began the process of becoming a client.

Lessons Learned

Be aware that caregivers also get sick.

Caregivers are not the indestructible, invulnerable people we think we are. Bad things can and do happen. Keep an active, updated file of pertinent information in case you are incapacitated and someone must step in. Include a list of your care responsibilities and daily medications, organized by time of day, the name of your stroke survivor's primary care physician, and copies of corresponding insurance cards arranged in a small three-ring notebook. Put this information in a prominent place familiar to both your stroke survivor and respite-care worker.

Choose the people to contact immediately if you become ill.

Keep a list of telephone numbers for family members, close friends, and physicians whom you can contact day or night for help. Make the list easily reachable in case of an emergency – in your wallet, on your night table, and on the speed dial of your cell phone. Be sure these people have a house key in case you cannot open the door yourself. Also let several neighbors know where you hide your emergency key.

Develop an emergency-support plan.

Personal emergencies are unscheduled and can upset the best of intentions. Work out your plan on paper with directions, medications, schedule, appointments, and key people to be notified if you are ill. Add this plan to your medical binder as a guide when you are away. Discuss the plan with people on your list.

Plan for the worst.

Make long-term-care plans for your stroke survivor in the event that you become seriously ill or even die. Choose a care facility and file the necessary forms so that you've established a record in case you are unable to do so later. However, because these facilities operate on a space-available basis, be aware that they may not have a vacancy during your emergency. Prepare and freeze extra meals to cover several days. Also maintain several extra days' worth of medications in your pill container.

Chapter 18

One Stroke, Two Survivors

Men and Women Were Created to Go through Life Two by Two

Sometimes people will ask me why I've fought so hard to reclaim Herb's mind and spirit. That is an easy question to answer. I have loved Herb since the day I met him, even though he was then and still is irascible and stubborn. From the beginning, Herb and I formed a combustible team. What brought us together despite our hardheadedness was an insatiable intellectual curiosity, similar frame of values, and mutual attraction.

Trust and challenge have long formed the wellspring from which we draw our strength. If Herb and I had not shared such an intense relationship, I doubt whether we would have had the emotional ferocity separately and together to claw our way to post-stroke survival.

We have been blessed with a long marriage, successful business careers, three wonderful adult children, and four amazing grandchildren. In our naïveté we fully expected to continue along our merry way, enriching the rest of our lives with work, grandparenting, and travel. Herb's massive stroke abruptly ended a comfortable transition to our so-called "golden years." With his catastrophic illness, our lives turned upside down and inside out. From my perspective, in addition to collecting a boatload of responsibilities, I lost my best friend, my husband, and my lover.

Life will never be the same as it was before the stroke. Our combustible tempers spawn many arguments, especially over my demands that

Herb push more physically rather than passively watch television. I don't see my husband as less of a man than he was before. While he may be physically limited, his mind functions well, and I refuse to allow him to succumb to self-pity. The going is tough for both of us.

Gradually, with encouragement from our rehab psychologist, we've talked through mutual needs and discovered that we both strive to reclaim intimacy and our special connection. It feels reassuring and wonderful to once again bed down sharing the warmth of our bodies. Perhaps more will come as recovery becomes easier.

Lessons Learned

Understand the link between depression and loss of sexual interest.

Both the caregiver and the stroke survivor can lose interest in activities that they once shared, including sex. Decreased energy, fatigue, and burnout are symptoms of both depression and exhaustion.

Seek outside professional support.

Look to your rehab psychologist or internist for insights and support as you wrestle with sexual doubts and perhaps even a fraying personal relationship. Supportive counsel allows you to air frustrations and clarify hidden thoughts.

Value the stroke survivor's needs.

It is critically important to talk through and share your differing perspectives. Even with few words and limited actions, search for those areas that can restore intimacy, warmth, and perspective.

Resume slowly and mutually.

Both of you need to feel comfortable and willing to reach out to each other. Whatever the physical limitations, you can find ways to share warmth and love.

Chapter 19
Restoring Self-Reliance
As Long as an Inchworm Moves Forward, It Progresses

Before his massive stroke, Herb lived a vital, intellectually challenging life and felt in control of his destiny. Overnight, and seemingly without obvious pain or discomfort, the stroke stripped away everything that in his view made him a man. This huge inability to walk, talk, drive a car, and care for his most basic needs rocked him down to his core.

From the beginning, in order to evaluate Herb's progress, it was important to combat his passivity with concrete, measurable tasks. Conservatively ramped up, the tasks proceeded through increasingly higher levels of complexity. Goal-setting has become part of my life. While it is unrealistic to expect that Herb will again mow the lawn, cut the hedges, or remove the storm windows, he can and will do more as the years advance. We have much further to go in our recovery journey.

Herb accepts change reluctantly. Independent dressing still prompts occasional tears of frustration from both of us. The process is tedious and I prefer not to watch. Except for his heavy shoes, Herb now dresses himself. Undressing is another matter.

Perhaps the biggest breakthrough of all is his ability to handle the urinal and free me of a less appealing responsibility. Now I can disappear for an hour or two, either into a different room or away from the house. We haven't reached the point where Herb will roll himself over to the refrigerator and prepare his own lunch. But he didn't do that before his stroke. Of all the possible tasks, this one remains the least probable.

Herb's speech has improved significantly. At least 90 percent of what he says either in direct conversation or over the telephone is intelligible. He willingly engages in conversation across the dinner table and voices opinions about current events.

The stroke disrupted both our lives and wishing won't make it go away. But we are learning to adapt and extend Herb's limitations as much as possible. An overall routine has set in as we get on with our lives. Even hard tasks are easier now that they are better established. We still have plenty of life, interest, and curiosity to find a satisfying life after stroke. My job as wife and caregiver is to make sure we stretch the long term even longer.

Lessons learned

Set goals.

Goal-setting is valuable because it leaves a measurable trail. You know where you are going because you build on where you have been.

You can't save someone who doesn't want to be saved.

You can fight for your loved one, slay dragons, battle the medical and insurance establishments, and handle all the daily necessities. But unless your stroke patient can conquer depression and is willing to move forward, you'll find yourselves spinning in circles. The effort has to be shared. If not, the caregiver must learn to walk away, emotionally as well as physically. That is truly tough love.

Fight for life and wellness.

It doesn't come automatically. Most survivors will probably seek the easiest way and simply live on a day-to-day basis. They need a push.

Search for pilot therapy programs.

If you live near a medical school or teaching hospital, or are a veteran, check with these institutions' stroke departments to see whether they offer studies in which your survivor might participate. Also search the Internet.

Seek cultural programs with matinee performances.

As you make your way back into the world, find programs that are conducive to your schedule and achievable without great stress. Matinees offer afternoon performances and daytime driving.

Return autonomy to your stroke survivor.

Hovering and helping too much aren't good for either the stroke survivor or the caregiver. The return of power, decision, and responsibility is very tough, but necessary for both. You must learn to let go.

Don't feel you have to follow all the advice that professionals offer.

Value your own judgment and common sense. Adapt those suggestions that work for you in your situation. Discard the others.

Chapter 20
Conclusion
There Is No Vision as Perfect as Hindsight

Nothing in our previous lives prepared us for the challenges of cataclysmic illness. Caught in the grip of stroke, Herb and I searched for strength in one another and in a higher power with a capacity greater than ours. I believed from the beginning that Herb could and would improve. While the stroke might ravage his body, I pledged that it would not destroy his mind and spirit. My toughest job has been to convince him to push forward despite all the obvious obstacles.

As I see my husband slowly but steadily reemerging, my confidence increases that sometime in the future I may yet regain my companion and best friend. This awareness sweeps away all the hard work and doubts that preceded it. There will always be shadows, because a survivor requires great vigilance to guard against another stroke. With steady, hard work, we've learned that incremental improvements lead to larger ones. We are fortunate to build on a foundation of forty-plus years of shared obstinacy and willpower along with mutual trust, respect, and love. These fundamentals are forged even stronger today. The strength of our relationship fuels the engine for even greater recovery.

We have learned many hard and humbling lessons in our journey back to the world of the living. The most profound of these is our realization that at no time, even at points of our greatest despair, did we struggle alone or in isolation. More than our own efforts, we have benefited from the support, kindness, and wisdom of so many others who surround us.

Lessons Learned

Survival builds on hope, stamina on progress.

You can't give up.

Recovery requires a cosmos.

A vast community of resources, love, and support buoys our own small efforts.

Acknowledgments:
Key Participants in Our Journey

We have many people to thank for their strength and support on our difficult journey. We begin with our family: our daughters and son, Kathryn, Miriam, and Steve Kleiman; our niece Anne Kleiman; William and Thérèse Kleiman, Herb's brother and our sister-in-law; Alan and Lois Elkin, Berenice's brother and our sister-in-law.

Our home crew provided inspiration and support: Sara Kass, "surrogate" daughter, trainer, friend; Otis Bush, respite caregiver and friend; Anna Debrogorski, home physical therapist; John Lee, t'ai chi instructor; Deborah Lief, trainer; Henry Miles, handyman and craftsman in charge of all things that need fixing; and Conor Willis, dog-walker extraordinaire. We deeply appreciate the sage financial guidance provided by our accountant, Joyce Graham, and our broker, Don Jacobson.

We are grateful to family, friends, and professionals who read rough drafts of our *One Stroke, Two Survivors* manuscript and shared comments and critiques: Laurie and Aaron Billowitz; Elizabeth Dreben; Susan Golden; Kathy Grekco; Mary Jo Ely; Miriam Kleiman; Ethel Morrison; Bill Pitts, founder of the Cleveland Stroke Club; Tena Rosner; Maxine Schinagle; Eran Shiloh; Naomi Soifer; and Alan Weiss. Michael Felver wrote the foreword and provided editorial support and medical terminology.

Marc Golub generously donated his time and expertise to establish our website, www.onestroketwosurvivors.com, and provided photography, digital scanning, and retouching. Beth Brumbaugh and Greg Hackett thoughtfully contributed the treadmill that keeps Herb moving forward.

We extend special thanks to the professionals we hold in good standing for reaching beyond the minimum and pulling us through some very difficult problems: Miriam Cohen, MD, Heart Associates Inc. at Union Memorial Hospital, Baltimore; Elizabeth Dreben, PhD, Rehabilitation Psychologist, MetroHealth Medical Center; Michael Felver, MD, Dept. of Internal Medicine, Cleveland Clinic Foundation; Michael Frankel, MD, Gastroenterology Associates of Cleveland; Brian Garrity, PT, the Claude D. Pepper Center, Geriatric Research Education Clinical Center, University of Maryland; Andrew P. Goldberg, MD, Professor of Medicine at the University of Maryland School of Medicine and Director of the Claude D. Pepper Older Americans Independence Center; Karen Kahn, DDS, Dept. of Dentistry, Cleveland Clinic Foundation; Anne Kleiman, DO, Associate Attending of Neurology, Metropolitan Hospital, NYC; Richard Macko, MD, Associate Professor of Neurology at the University of Maryland School of Medicine and director of the stroke progress program at the Baltimore VA; Asikin Mentari, MD, Dept. of Rehabilitation, MetroHealth Medical Center; Kathleen Michael, PhD, RN, CRRN, Program Manager, the Claude D. Pepper Center, Geriatric Research Education Clinical Center, University of Maryland; Peter Rasmussen, MD, Dept. of Neurosurgery, Cleveland Clinic Foundation; David Sholitan, MD, Dept. of Ophthalmology, Cleveland Clinic Foundation; Jill Whitall, PhD, Associate Professor of Physical Therapy at the University of Maryland School of Medicine and stroke progress program leader; Nishan Tambay, MD, formerly of the Dept. of Rehabilitation, MetroHealth Medical Center; Alan Weiss, MD, Dept. of Internal Medicine, Cleveland Clinic Foundation.

And I reserve special thoughts for my toughest critic, guide, manuscript editor, and graphic designer, Steve Kleiman.

Appendix 1
Words to Know

Charcot-Marie-Tooth disease	A progressive neuromuscular disorder that mainly affects the limbs.
cholesterol	A form of blood fat that may settle into artery walls.
diabetes	A chronic disease marked by high levels of sugar in the blood.
Hb A1c	A test that measures the amount of glycosylated hemoglobin in the blood. The test gives a good estimate of how well diabetes is being managed over time.
HDL	*High-density lipoprotein.* The "good" cholesterol, best if above 50.
hematocrit	The percentage of whole blood composed of red blood cells.
hematoma	An accumulation of blood in tissue, usually caused by trauma.
hemiparesis	Using only one side of the body because the other side has been weakened by stroke.

LDL	*Low-density lipoprotein.* The "bad" cholesterol, except if below 100.
lipid (a)	A lipoprotein associated with vascular damage; may be genetically linked.
lipid profile	A measure of the level of various fats in the blood.
Medicare Part A	Medicare coverage for inpatient costs in hospitals and skilled nursing facilities.
Medicare Part B	Medicare coverage of physician services, outpatient hospital care, and some other medical services that Part A does not cover.
MRA	*Magnetic resonance angiogram.* An MRI procedure that assesses the patterning of intracranial vessels and whether arteries inside the skull are clogged.
MRI	*Magnetic resonance imaging.* A noninvasive procedure that uses powerful magnets and radio waves and is particularly useful for the brain. The patient is asked to lie on a narrow table which slides into a large tunnel-like tube within the scanner.
OT	Occupational therapists help people improve their basic motor functions and perform tasks in daily living and working environments.

PT	Physical therapists help restore function, improve mobility, relieve pain, and prevent or limit permanent physical disabilities of patients suffering from injuries or disease.
ST	Speech therapists help people with speech problems to shape thoughts and communicate ideas into words.
stroke	An interruption of the blood supply to any part of the brain, resulting in damaged brain tissue. Stroke is the third leading cause of death in most developed countries and the leading cause of disability in adults. Most strokes are due to blood clots that block blood flow.
TIA	*Transient ischemic attack.* Caused by an interruption of blood flow to brain cells, it results in strokelike symptoms that resolve within 24 hours. If the symptoms do not resolve completely, the event is called a stroke.
tPA	*Tissue plasminogen activator.* Injected intravenously, it activates enzymes that can dissolve a blood clot in an hour or two; if tPA is given within the first two to three hours of stroke onset, it may reduce permanent disability; in rare cases, the treatment may result in internal bleeding.

Appendix 2

Useful Resources on the Internet

There is excellent information about stroke-related issues available from worldwide resources on the Internet. The following well-documented websites are useful, but I urge caution in your searches because abundant misinformation circulates on the Web. Corroborate information with established medical and governmental sites. Because caregivers have little time or inclination for research, you may want to ask others to conduct the search for you. Here are a few sites I think are worthwhile.

One Stroke, Two Survivors **website**
> www.onestroketwosurvivors.com
> A working guide for stroke survivors

The Cleveland Clinic
> www.clevelandclinic.org/health
> Provides a broad range of health support

National Stroke Association
> www.stroke.org
> Lists studies, breakthroughs

American Stroke Association
> www.strokeassociation.org
> Includes programs, care, caregivers' support

The Stroke Network
> www.strokenetwork.org
> An online support group with message board and chat room

National Institutes of Health/National Institute of Neurological
Disorders and Stroke (NINDS)
www.ninds.nih.gov/disorders/stroke/stroke.htm
Basic details about stroke

Internet Stroke Center at Washington University in St. Louis
www.strokecenter.org/education/rx_complications/2.html
Preventing and managing stroke complications

Depression and Stroke
www.nimh.nih.gov/publicat/depstroke.cfm
Depression as one of the major complications of stroke

Rehabilitation and Stroke
www.ninds.nih.gov/disorders/stroke/stroke.htm
www.arni.uk.com
Rehabilitation programs and expectations

Chronic Pain after Stroke
http://www.painrelieffoundation.org.uk/paininfo/paininfo_
cpsp.html
Good background reading

Complications of Diabetes and Stroke
http://my.webmd.com/context/article/46/1667_50942.htm
Good background reading

Complications of Stroke
www.wrongdiagnosis.com/s/stroke/complic.htm
Good background reading

Pharmaceutical Support
www.rxassist.org or www.needymeds.com
Special pharmaceutical programs

Canadian Drugstore
www.rxnorth.com
Ordering online from RxNorth

Stroke Caregivers Handbook
www.strokesafe.org/Handbook.html
Information for caregivers

Caregiver's Bill of Rights
www.mindspring.com/~tscotent/bill.htm
What to expect and demand in proper care

Appendix 3

Herbert S. Kleiman Daily Medications (3/2/04)

Here is one of the prepared information sheets we bring to medical and dental appointments. Information compiled on one sheet is an efficient way to avoid giving the first fifteen minutes of an appointment to discussing and recording medications. I find this tool valuable and rely on its accuracy when I fill Herb's medicine boxes every two weeks because it lists medications, dosages, time of day, and name of prescribing physician (for new medications).

8:00 AM

Pills

Plavix	1	75 mg per Dr. D. Hammer 1/03
Metoprolol (Lopressor)	1/2	25 mg
Glyburide	1	@ 5 mg
Metformin (Glucophage)	1	850 mg
Lisinopril (Zestril)	1/2	@ 5 mg
Nitroglycerin capsule	1	6.5 mg per Dr. M. Cohen, 5/2/02
MiraLax	daily	1 measured capful
Celexa	1	40 mg per Dr. Weiss 6/2/03
Centrum Silver vitamin	1	Per Dr. Weiss

Inhalation

Advair Diskus	1 spray	100/50

4:00 – 6:00 PM _____

Pills

Nitroglycerin capsule	1	6.5 mg per Dr. M. Cohen, 5/2/02
Glyburide	1/2	@ 2.5 mg
Tricor	1 every other day	54 mg Per Dr. Sprecher, 4/15/02 per Dr. Cohen, 1/04
Foltx sf/df	1	25 mg folic acid
Cozaar	1	25 mg per Dr. Cohen, 1/04
Aspirin	1	81 mg/coated aspirin

9:00 – 10:00 PM _____

Pills

Metoprolol (Lopressor)	1/2	25 mg
Trazodone	1	100 mg as needed for sleep

Inhalation

Advair Diskus	1 spray	100/50

Appendix 4

Herbert S. Kleiman Summary Sheet (10/2/02)

Here is one of our prepared information sheets from Herb's loose-leaf medical file that I carry on trips and distribute at all new medical and therapy appointments. A medical history at one glance avoids lots of repetitive questions. I also keep a separate file for my own records.

Patient's Comprehensive Medical History

- Charcot-Marie-Tooth disease (since childhood but diagnosed in 1973)

- Type 2 diabetes mellitus, diagnosed in 1983

- Asthma, diagnosed in 1977

- Hypercholesterolemia

- Stroke-related severe right hemiparesis re 7/14/01

- Stents (2) arteriosclerosis re 3/18/02

- Transfusions (2) re iron deficiency anemia on 5/10/02

- Speech prosthesis with pharyngeal wax; consult and initial steps begun 2/26; monthly buildup through Sept. 13, 2002; prosthesis discontinued at that time. NO PRIOR FACIAL PAIN.

- FACIAL PAIN begins approximately mid-September 2002; panoramic film by Cleveland Clinic dentistry dept. on 9/25/02 indicates no dental pathology.

- Subsequent visits and assessments with 3 Cleveland Clinic neurologists, including a specialist in trigeminal neuralgia; 3 dentists including general, periodontist, endodontist (2 unrelated root-canals); Cleveland Clinic Pain Center including a nerve block; 4 sets of acupuncture through MetroHealth Medical Center. Neurontin and Trileptal found to offer no benefit. No diagnosis other than atypical facial pain.

- Pain continues and ranges on scale from 1- 8 with increasing intensity over last 4 months.

Recent Stroke History

7/14/01	Patient has first stroke. Admitted to Cleveland Clinic.
7/17/01	Worsening of right hemiparesis and dysarthria: emergency angiography.
7/17/01	Stents inserted into carotid and left middle cerebral arteries.
7/26/01	Patient transferred to MetroHealth Stroke Rehabilitation acute care.
8/28/01	Discharged from MetroHealth Hospital to home.
9/4/01- 10/1/01	North Coast home nursing care including nursing, physical, occupational, and speech (minimal) therapies.
9/11/01	Cleveland Clinic emergency room visit due to muscular spasms in arms and pain in left shoulder. Demonstrated emotional distress related to national calamity on this day. Examination reveals no heart problem, but a urinary tract infection. Patient is discharged without overnight stay, with prescription for Bactrim.

9/14/01	Cleveland Clinic emergency room visit due to dehydration and exhaustion. Patient admitted for one-night observation and extensive blood/ultrasound testing. Prescription changed to Cipro.
9/18/01	Patient passes modified barium swallow study (4th effort) and is advised to receive ENT evaluation for suspected vocal cord paralysis.
10/02/01	Patient begins outpatient therapy at MetroHealth Stroke Rehabilitation Center.
3/18/02	Cardiac angioplasty with 2 stents at Cleveland Clinic.

Medications (3/16/07)

Here is a shortened listing of Herb's medications, which I update before each medical visit. This concise list of medications and dosages offers both a safety mechanism and a brief summary at a certain point in recovery.

Plavix	75 mg
Metoprolol	25 mg (1/2 tablet 2x)
Glyburide	5 mg tablet (1 1/2x per day)
Glucophage	850 mg tablet
Nitroglycerin	6.5 mg capsule (2x per day)
Celexa	40 mg tablet
Lisinopril	10 mg tablet (1/2 per day)
Aspirin	81 mg tablet
Trazodone	100 mg tablet (1/2 per day)
Advair Diskus	100/50 (1 spray 2x)
Tricor	54 mg (every other day)
Foltx	25 mg folic acid
MiraLax	1 capful daily
Centrum Silver	1 daily

Appendix 6

Memo of 5/18/02 to Physician Team

Frustrated that the many specialists did not communicate with one another and/or appeared unaware of Herb's multiple complications, I devised this summary memo. My bottom line was that I required each physician on this list to send all subsequent reports, tests, and memos to our internist and me.

Re: Patient – Herbert S. Kleiman (Clinic #; MHC #; Soc. Sec. #)

To: Drs. (listed by name, phone number, and fax)

Subject: Coordination and Communication

We are fortunate to have a health-care team of wonderful, very caring professionals and friends who are working to establish a higher quality of life for Herb Kleiman, following his stroke on July 14, 2001, and stenting in mid-March 2002. You represent four different hospital systems within two states. In an attempt to update Herb's records, improve communication, and avoid duplication of effort, please note the following:

• Dr. Alan Weiss, listed above, has replaced Dr. Michael Felver as Herb's internist and team coordinator, effective immediately. *All procedures, blood tests, and results should go through Dr. Weiss with copies to me.* Dr. Felver, who has an aggressive travel schedule, has kindly agreed to remain as an adviser.

• Dr. Miriam Cohen, cardiologist, Union Memorial Hospital in Baltimore, provided a second opinion in late April. She performed a Persantine nuclear stress test. A summary including corresponding blood work is available through Dr. Weiss (or me). The result:

although there is diffuse ASCVD with severe 3-vessel coronary artery disease – with stents in the RCA and LAD, the situation is now stabilized. Because of Herb's many medical problems and the fact that he is virtually asymptomatic from a cardiac standpoint at this time, medical management rather than bypass surgery should be optimized and continued.

- Of concern, however, were both a hematocrit of 28 with 6 percent iron saturation, which indicates slow blood loss, and a white count of 13,000. Dr. Cohen recommended that Herb be seen immediately by both his urologist and gastroenterologist. She further prescribed a long-acting nitro capsule, 6.5 mg b.i.d., 2 x per day and recommended that he have another Persantine nuclear stress test in 4-6 months, depending on his clinical status.

- Dr. Michael Frankel, gastroenterologist, reviewed Dr. Cohen's analysis. Prior to initiating both endoscopic and colonoscopic procedures, he arranged for the transfusion of 2 units of blood on May 10, 2002, at Hillcrest Hospital, and began a series of 16 iron injections (2 per week for 8 weeks).

- Dr. Martin Resnick cultured Herb's urine and on May 16 reported evidence of gram-positive bacteria, with >100,000 colonies of Group D strep, nonenterococcus. He prescribed ampicillin, 250 mg, for 10 days followed by a second culture.

- Dr. Weiss assumed management of Herb's case on May 13. He has reviewed all past records, including Dr. Cohen's results, and added chronic sinusitis to the lengthy list of ailments. He prescribed Flonase 0.05 percent nasal spray (one puff per 1x per day) – and recommended eliminating Actos, Ditropan, and Remeron from Herb's list of meds.

- Dr. John Perl II, endovascular neurosurgery, ordered a follow-up CAT scan to monitor any repeating stenosis of the brain. This was conducted yesterday, 5/17 at the Clinic along with a CBC. He will issue a report on Monday, May 20. Dr. Perl will be moving out of state at the end of May and will refer Herb to a successor.

That sums up activity for the past two weeks. Please, folks, it is absolutely necessary that specialist members of this team coordinate with Dr. Weiss, confer with one another, and share results and perhaps conflicts before overlapping. Telephone and fax numbers are provided above. I further require copies of all written records faxed to me at (phone #) as a fail-safe.

Again, Herb and I thank all of you from the bottom of our hearts for reaching out and performing such Herculean efforts not only to keep him alive but in hope of achieving continuing progress.

Sincerely,

Berenice Kleiman

Suggested Readings

There are few available and inspiring books about stroke survivors from a firsthand perspective. Bauby's *The Diving Bell and the Butterfly* is particularly poignant and inspirational because it is written by a paralyzed stroke victim who could move only one eye. He died one day before his book was published. Also included on my list is a variety of books that provide background and support.

Jean-Dominique Bauby. *The Diving Bell and the Butterfly: A Memoir of Life in Death.* New York: Knopf, 1997.

Rosalynn Carter, with Susan K. Golant. *Helping Someone with Mental Illness: A Compassionate Guide for Family, Friends, and Caregivers.* New York: Crown, 1998.

Kenneth J. Doka. *Living with Life-Threatening Illness: A Guide for Patients, Their Families, and Caregivers.* New York: Lexington Books, 1993.

Susan Edsall. *Into the Blue: A Father's Flight and a Daughter's Return.* New York: St. Martin's Press, 2004.

Arthur Josephs. *The Invaluable Guide to Life after Stroke: An Owner's Manual.* Long Beach, CA: Amadeus Press, 1992.

Robert McCrum. *My Year Off: Recovering Life after a Stroke.* New York: W. W. Norton, 1998.

Kristine Napier. *Eat Away Diabetes: Beat Type 2 Diabetes by Winning the Blood Sugar Battle.* New York: Prentice Hall Press, 2002.

Dean Ornish. *Dr. Dean Ornish's Program for Reversing Heart Disease: The Only System Scientifically Proven to Reverse Heart Disease Without Drugs or Surgery.* New York: Ballantine Books, 1995.

————. *Everyday Cooking with Dr. Dean Ornish: 150 Easy, Low-Fat, High-Flavor Recipes.* New York: HarperCollins, 2002.

Ellen Paullin. *Ted's Stroke: The Caregiver's Story.* Cabin John, MD: Seven Locks Press, 1988.

Richard C. Senelick, Peter W. Rossi, and Karla Dougherty. *Living with Stroke: A Guide for Families.* 3rd ed. Chicago: Contemporary Books, 2001.

Artemis P. Simopoulos and Jo Robinson. *The Omega Diet: The Life-saving Nutritional Program Based on the Diet of the Island of Crete.* New York: HarperCollins, 1999.

Index

A

accessibility
    home evaluation, 19
    of restaurants versus friends' homes, 59
accounting software, 74-75
adult incontinence products, 66-67
accessibility
    home evaluation, 19
    of restaurants versus friends' homes, 59
accounting software, 74-75
adult incontinence products, 66-67
accounting software, 74-75
advocacy
    for improvements to public facilities, 67
    for stroke patient, 12-13, 44-45
age at time of stroke, 1
American Association of Retired Persons (AARP), 73
anger management, 47-50
applesauce, 29
appointments
    bundling, 45
    lightweight transit chair for, 26
    preparing for, 39, 41, 45

B

baby monitors, 23
backpack for toileting products, 27, 67
balance problems as sign of stroke, 10
bench with a side handle, 32-33
blood clot stroke, 10
blood vessel bursting stroke, 10
board certification, 37
body wash, no-rinse, 29
brain damage, prompt action versus, 2, 9
burnout prevention, 31-33, 47-50
business card file, 45

C

D

E

emergency call buttons, positioning of, 17-18
emergency medical services (EMS), 2-3, 11
emergency-support plan, 83
equipment
    at home, 22-23
    urinals, 27, 65, 89
    wheelchair, 25-27
exercise
    for caregiver, 27-28, 49
    increasing blood flow with, 53
    for stroke patient, 5, 52-54
expenses, 73-76
experimental programs, 54-55

F

falls of stroke patient, 31-33
family history and stroke, 2
family support, 12, 28, 57-59. *See also caregivers*
fiber, 63
finances, 73-76
food-smart recovery, 61-63
friends' support, 57-59
friends' visits, 32, 58-59
functional mobility, developing, 17, 33, 52, 99

G

generic medications, 78
genetics and stroke, 2
goal setting, 89-91
grocery shopping, 63
ground rules for visitors, 58
guilt, 50

H

handicap-accessible hotel accommodations, 69-71
Hb A1c, 97
HDL cholesterol, 97

headaches, severe, as sign of stroke, 10
health insurance, 73-75
hematocrit, 97, 114
hematoma, 97
hemiparesis, 97
high blood sugar, 61-62, 97
home
    practicing therapies at, 52, 54
    preparing, 21-22
home accessibility evaluation, 19
home care by agency, limitations of, 25, 28
home team, selecting and training, 31-33
hospitals
    atmosphere in, 15-16
    expertise in stroke at, 2-3, 11
    itemized statements from, 75-76
hospital social workers, 15-16
hotel accommodations, 69-71

I
illness of caregiver, 81-83
incontinence products, 66-67
insurance policies
    health and long-term care, 73-75
    understanding coverage, 26
Internet research, 4, 38, 101-103
IRS deductions, 74-75

# L
LDL cholesterol, 98
lipid (a), 98
lipid profile, 98
living wills, 75
long-term-care insurance, 73-75

M
magnetic resonance angiograph (MRA), 98
magnetic resonance imaging (MRI), 98

N

neighbors, help from, 57-58
911 calls, 11
notebook, 13. *See also medical binder*
numbness as sign of stroke, 10
nursing care
    home nursing services, 22, 25, 28, 82
    in rehab facility, 17
nursing home solution, indicators for, 4
nutritionists, 62

O

occupational therapists (OTs), 17, 52, 99
one-sided pyramid walker, 5, 25, 32
outpatient rehab therapy, 28, 51-53
outpatient therapy, 51-55

P

pain, 38
paralysis as sign of stroke, 10
patient-assistance programs (PAPs), 80
Patient Prescription Information (PPI), 41
Patient's Bill of Rights, 19
Persantine nuclear stress test, 113-114
pharmaceuticals. *See medications*
physical therapists (PTs), 17, 33, 52, 99
pill organizers, 23
pilot therapy programs, 91
plateau, 51, 54
power-of-attorney documents, 75
prayer, asking for, 12
prepaid telephone cards, 12
priorities, 19
progress, uncertain nature of, 5
protective window, 11-12
psychologist, need for, 17, 19, 86
pyramid walker, 5, 25, 32
See also one-sided pyramid walker